SAVE A LIFE

GW00502365

SAVE
—A—
LIFE

JUDITH FISHER
ANDREW MARSDEN
JENNY ROGERS

BBC PUBLICATIONS

This book accompanies the BBC Television series
Save A Life first broadcast on BBC 1 from October
1986, produced by Jenny Rogers and Julian
Stenhouse.

The HEC student booklet text on pages 117–134
reproduced by kind permission of the Health
Education Council, London

Front cover illustration by Cathie Felstead
Diagrams by Will Giles
Charts by Oxford Illustrators Ltd

Published to accompany a series of programmes
prepared in consultation with the
BBC Continuing Education Advisory Council

© The Authors and BBC Enterprises Limited 1986
First published 1986

Published by BBC Publications,
a division of BBC Enterprises Ltd,
35 Marylebone High Street, London W1M 4AA

ISBN 0 563 21277 2

This book is set in 10/11 Plantin Light Monophoto

Typeset by Ace Filmsetting Ltd, Frome, Somerset
Printed in England by Cox & Wyman Ltd, Reading
Cover printed by Malvern Press Ltd, London, England

CONTENTS

About the Authors

Judith Fisher MBBS, MRCGP is a General Practitioner in East London and Honorary Secretary of the British Association for Immediate Care (BASICS) and was founder-Chairman of the Resuscitation Council (UK), a group of distinguished doctors devoted to setting national standards where resuscitation is concerned.

Andrew Marsden MB, ChB, FRCS(Ed) is Consultant in Accident and Emergency Medicine at Pinderfields Hospital, Wakefield. He started the Wakefield Life Support Scheme which, in a short time, has already trained 5000 members of the public in emergency aid. He is Chairman of the Resuscitation Council.

Jenny Rogers BA is a Senior Producer in the BBC's Continuing Education Television Department, and produced the *Save A Life* television programmes. Before becoming a producer she worked in adult education, first as a teacher, then as a BBC Education Officer. Her books on teaching adults are widely regarded as standard works on the subject.

INTRODUCTION

Every year in the United Kingdom about 60 000 people die suddenly, prematurely and unexpectedly. At a rough estimate, up to one third of these sudden deaths could be averted if the right help were given promptly. That's 20 000 lives saved each year. The role of the ordinary citizen in emergency life support is grossly underestimated. Many cases of sudden death – for example, from drowning or following unconsciousness – may be caused by very simple things, such as airway obstruction from a 'floppy' tongue. They can be prevented by carrying out basic first aid manoeuvres, manoeuvres which can be taught to everyone. What's more, most sudden deaths occur in the home or when a relative is present. Family members are well motivated to respond to crisis – they simply need to know what to do. This is why the national *Save A Life* campaign is being mounted to teach the public the rudiments of resuscitation and emergency aid. It is the aim of this book to provide answers to the questions 'What should be taught?' and 'How should we teach it?'.

The idea of having a campaign for mass education in emergency aid is not a new one, and we can learn much by looking at the efforts of those areas which have been running similar programmes for some time: Scandinavia, Holland, West Germany, Australasia and, especially, North America and Canada. The pioneering work from Seattle, a coastal town in the American north west, deserves a special mention. There, heart specialist Dr Leonard Cobb realised that the problem of sudden death from heart disease was essentially a pre-hospital problem. He therefore set up a programme called 'Medic I', in which paramedics were trained and equipped to give advanced technical assistance to people outside hospital, mainly through using a 'defibrillator', a machine which can shock back into life a heart that has stopped.

Cobb's programme proved very successful and many lives have been saved because of it. But the success rate for defibrillation depends on how quickly the machine can be used and the longer the brain remains without oxygen the less chance there is that the victim will recover. So Seattle began an interesting experiment: 'Medic II'. A campaign was mounted to train the community in those essential life-saving steps which we have come to speak of as cardiopulmonary (heart-lung) resuscitation, or CPR for short. By 1985, 350 000 citizens (almost half of the population) had received training in the three-hour 'Heartsaver' course. Within the first ten years the rate of successful resuscitation in the city has doubled and not only for cases of heart disease – sudden deaths from drowning, poisoning, electric shock and road accidents are being prevented as well. The amount of training given and the quality of CPR performed seems to be unrelated to outcome. Apparently it's better for a lot of people to know a little than for a few to learn a lot.

Emergency first aid is now part of the American high school curriculum, and a recent Gallup poll has revealed that one in five Americans are familiar with CPR procedures. There is little doubt that it is partly because of this success of the CPR campaigns that the incidence of sudden death from heart disease in the United States is falling.

In Britain, too, community resuscitation schemes have been introduced – sixteen by January 1986. The first was Dr Chamberlain's Heart Guard campaign in Brighton which was set up in 1978. Within the first five years 25 000 citizens had received training and 46 lives had been saved as a result, 16 solely and wholly through intervention by members of the public. In the first year of its existence, the Life Support Training Scheme in Wakefield trained 5000 people with five lives saved.

The cost of this work is no more than £5000 capital and £1 per head training charges. The move now to establish more such schemes to educate the general public in CPR does not imply criticism of the existing health services. The aim is simply to increase our health care through involvement of the whole community.

HOW TO USE THIS BOOK

You will not need any prior medical knowledge in order to follow this book, but it is primarily aimed at those who already train the general public in resuscitation techniques. You may be a lay instructor with one of the voluntary first aid societies, a member of one of the emergency services or the armed forces, a teacher, a health care professional or a well motivated layman. Probably you will already know the basic CPR and first aid procedures back to front. However, one problem even for experienced first-aid tutors is to know how to prune down this knowledge to fit a 2–3 hour training session. The *Save A Life* Campaign Coordinating Committee spent many anguished hours agreeing a basic curriculum that was both practical and appropriate. You will find this on p. 141. It is important to keep to this outline as a foundation as far as possible, but how you treat the material is up to you.

We have probably given you far more information than you could actually use in such a short session. However, all the common procedures are described, together with a discussion of their underlying scientific basis. We have included some of the many questions we find are often asked at training sessions and the answers we typically give. We have also tried to anticipate some of the problem areas we find are highlighted by tutors.

Our guide can stand alone for anyone teaching emergency aid, but it also supplements the *Save A Life* Campaign booklet published by the HEC for students to take home from the training sessions. The text of this is printed in full on pp. 117-134. The booklet and this book are closely related to the BBC TV *Save A Life* programmes which are available on videotape (for details, see p. 147) and can be used in classes.

This book is not intended to replace the first-aid training manuals already available. We have written it simply as a source book of up-to-date thinking on resuscitation, together with some constructive ideas on how to put the information across. We have made every effort to reflect current practice, to accept the consensus of the *Save A Life* Coordinating Committee and to be non-controversial. Nevertheless there may be places where differences of opinion arise and consequently we emphasise here that the responsibility for the material in this book is ours and ours alone.

The *Save A Life* Campaign is one of the most exciting initiatives in community health education ever mounted in the UK. We hope you will enjoy being part of it as much as we enjoyed helping to plan it. Ultimately its success will depend entirely on your skill and enthusiasm in getting the information across to the general public. We hope this book will help you do it.

Judith Fisher, Andrew Marsden and Jenny Rogers

June 1986

THE CURRICULUM

BASICS

You must stress to your class at the start of the session that you are going to teach only those things which are vital in an emergency – more than this becomes part of the wider subject of First Aid.

We teach a simple ABC routine of resuscitation

A   Assess the situation: Are you in any danger your-self? Is the casualty conscious? Airway: Is the air-way open?

B   Breathing: Is the casualty breathing?

C   Circulation: Does the casualty have a pulse? Is the casualty bleeding?

The body can withstand lack of food for three weeks, lack of water for three days, but lack of air . . . ? After three to four minutes of oxygen starvation, brain

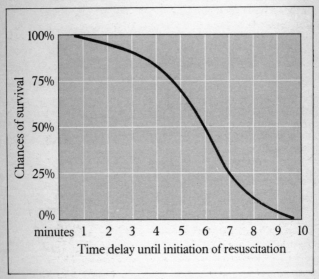

Diagram showing how soon chances of survival decrease if a cardiac arrest is not treated.

function will start to fail, the casualty will fall unconscious, breathing and heartbeats will cease and the casualty may die.

To get oxygen to the brain only three main body systems are involved. Explaining these briefly to your class is usually very helpful.

A Airway

This means the tubes connecting the atmosphere to the lungs. The airway is made up of: the air passages in the mouth and nose; the back of the mouth (pharynx); the voicebox (larynx); the windpipe (trachea) which lies in front of the gullet; and a network of pipes (the bronchi) leading to the air sacs in the lungs.

B Breathing

Breathing occurs when the muscles of the chest expand to allow air into the lungs and relax to let it out. In the lungs gases transfer from the air sacs to the blood stream. The air we breathe contains 20% oxygen and 80% nitrogen. We take in about one fifth of the oxygen present with each breath, exchanging this in the lungs for carbon dioxide. So the air we breathe out still contains 16% oxygen as well as 4% carbon dioxide, the

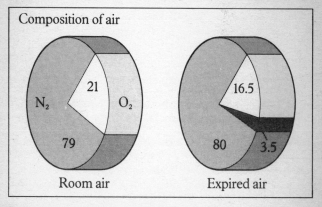

Percentage composition of room air and expired air.

nitrogen remaining unchanged. Breathing is controlled from the breathing centre of the brain; from this, nerves pass via the spinal cord to the chest muscles. Therefore breathing may stop not only as a result of problems within the chest but also from malfunction in the brain or paralysis to the spinal cord, spinal nerves or chest muscles.

C Circulation of the blood

This has two components:

A pump, ie the heart which rhythmically forces blood around the body 60–80 times per minute.

A set of pipes, ie the arteries and veins which conduct blood to and from all parts of the body including the brain. Just as with breathing, circulation is controlled from special centres in the brain and so may fail if the brain is damaged. The circulation may also fail because of heart damage (from a heart attack, for example) or from bleeding (haemorrhage), or the effects of shock.

Damage or blockage to the airway, a breakdown in the mechanism of breathing or a major fault in the circulation may mean the brain cannot get enough oxygen. Resuscitation is the name given to the technique used to overcome these situations. If the airway is blocked it must be opened; if breathing has stopped it must be re-started (usually by the rescuer breathing for the casualty in giving mouth-to-mouth ventilation); if there is no pulse this means the circulation around the body has stopped and the heart must be assisted by giving external chest compression. The combination of external chest compression and artificial ventilation is known as cardiopulmonary resuscitation or CPR.

Some common questions

Q Are there circumstances when people can live without breathing in which brain damage does not occur?

A Yes – in some cases of extreme cold (hypothermia) the brain's requirement for oxygen is reduced. (Use of this fact is made in some surgical operations.) There are examples on record of people – usually children – making a full recovery after having been rescued from relatively lengthy periods in cold water, with no breathing. On such occasions you must not presume death but carry on with mouth-to-mouth breathing as long as you are able, and ideally until after the body has warmed up to its normal temperature.

CALLING FOR HELP

Probably the most difficult thing for a lay person to assess is the need for help in any emergency. You must attempt to instil confidence and a sense of priorities into your students. They should always ask themselves 'Do I need help? If so from whom and why'. It may be that all that is needed is a neighbour or family friend with whom they can discuss the problem. It might be that the patient is known to his GP and this is a flare up of an existing disease, in which case the most appropriate person to call would be the family doctor. However, in most emergencies it is likely that an ambulance will be required. For instance, it has been shown in the USA that the earlier the emergency medical services are contacted, the higher the survival rate from heart attack. Encourage students to dial 999 and call for an ambulance in cases of:

> unconsciousness
> difficulty in breathing
> suspected heart attack
> severe bleeding
> serious burns

This is a useful time to discuss with the class how convenient it would be for a stranger to enter their home and get help to them quickly. Do they keep their own doctor's name and telephone number conspicuously by the telephone? Do they have their telephone number on their handset? (In these days of 'phone shops' many people purchase elaborate telephones but forget to put their own telephone number on the disc.) When the ambulance arrives can it find the house easily? Is there a large clear number on the gate and front door? Is there a porch light? Are there dustbins obstructing the pathway from the gate to the door? Do they live in a flat and, if so, is their name clearly displayed on a bell outside? Is their doorbell working?

Remind students there is no point in an ambulance responding rapidly only to have difficulty in finding the home. It is useful to tell everyone about the system used for emergency calls in this country. Protocols have been devised to make the whole process as speedy as possible. No money is required to make a 999 call from a public phone box. The numbers 999 were chosen as they are difficult to dial by accident but they are easy to feel with two fingers if you cannot see.

There will be two operators who will respond to a call. The first person is the emergency operator who will say, 'Emergency: which service are you calling?'. All the caller needs to say at this time is 'Ambulance Service, please'. He should listen to the operator and not rush in with a description of what has happened. This operator will then ring the ambulance service and while making this connection will ask him from which number he is calling. On receiving a reply from the ambulance service he will hear her say 'Ambulance, I am connecting you to [your number].' In these days of increasing vandalism it is useful to note that whereas the dial of a public phone box frequently does not have the number on it, both the number and situation of the box are also on a card sealed behind the small glass frame on the wall which often escapes damage.

Once connected to the ambulance service it is important that the caller gives succinct clear answers. Vague descriptions like 'Mr Hopkins next door has gone all breathless' sound much less urgent than 'my neighbour has choked on a piece of meat, he is unconscious, unable to breathe and not responding to back blows and finger sweeps'. In this sentence the caller has explained exactly what the emergency is and what treatment he has given. The ambulance service would consider this a sufficiently severe emergency to divert an ambulance to the scene even if it already has patients on board. They will not waste time suggesting the first aid measures of back blows and finger sweeps as these have already been tried. Remind students to speak slowly and calmly. The operator will have a list of questions that she needs to complete before she puts the handset down. A caller should never replace the telephone before the operator has said thank you and hung up. It is particularly important to give the exact site of the emergency and the number of patients. Callers could offer to send someone to the roadside or the nearest corner to direct the ambulance. If they are alone in a house with a casualty at night they could offer to open the front curtains and leave the lights on as it is difficult to spot houses in the dark. While the ambulance is being despatched the ambulance service may ask the caller if he wishes to give any form of emergency treatment. In Bristol the ambulance service will ask the caller if he wishes to give CPR and will take him step by step through the stages of resuscitation. It has already been shown in Seattle that this form of advice saves lives.

You will frequently be asked by your students whether they should also summon the fire service or police. Advise them that the severity of the accident will be gauged by the ambulance controller, who will send the other emergency vehicles if appropriate.

It is quite useful in your classes to act out such situations with one person playing the role of the panicky rescuer and the instructor acting as the telephone operator. Practising with your students will help them slow down and explain clearly what the problem has been. If you give them a scenario you can then help them to see what their priorities are and take them through this usually nerve-racking phase of emergency care.

A AIRWAY

A AIRWAY

You will probably find that while most students have heard of mouth-to-mouth breathing and chest compressions, very few realise the importance and simplicity of opening the airway. Explain that there are two main causes of airway obstruction:

a) The tongue

In an unconscious casualty the muscles go limp allowing the tongue to flop into the back of the throat. The base of the tongue closes off the airway so that no air can travel from the mouth or nose into the lungs. Unless the airway is opened again breathing will stop and circulation as well.

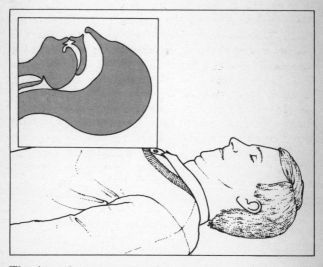

The airway in an unconconscious casualty.

b) *Foreign bodies*

'Intrinsic' foreign bodies are things which are caused by, or are part of the body, eg vomit, broken teeth, clots of blood, etc.

'Extrinsic' foreign bodies include displaced false teeth, pieces of undigested food, weeds in cases of drowning, and accidentally inhaled objects such as bits of toys and pens, etc. Advice for dealing with obstructing foreign bodies will be given in the section on choking (p. 51).

Opening the airway

Much of the experimental work to find the best means of opening the airway was carried out in the 1950s by the Drs Archer Gordon and James Elam. This work led to the description of the 'triple airway manoeuvre'

- Head tilt
- Chin lift
- Jaw thrust

Head tilt

Do stress that the most important action by far is tilting the head back to move the tongue forward away from the back of the throat. To perform 'head tilt', place the palm of one hand on the subject's forehead and tilt the

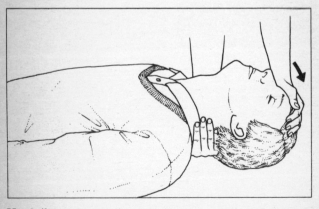

Head tilt.

head backwards as far as possible. The other hand should steady the neck – it is not necessary to 'lift' the neck upwards as was once taught, but simply to steady it during the tilting process.

Chin lift and jaw thrust

These manoeuvres are intended to overcome the sagging of the airway which a relaxed jaw causes in an unconscious casualty. Jaw thrust is an advanced technique, which if carried out incorrectly could result in dislocation of the jaw. It should *not* be shown to the general public. It is, however, possible to teach the chin lift or chin support, and this is a useful adjunct to the head tilt. To perform the chin lift, rescuers should place their fingers under the bony part of the casualty's chin and pull the chin upwards and forwards. With their fingers supporting the victim's chin they may be able to feel if there is any breathing against the palm of their hand.

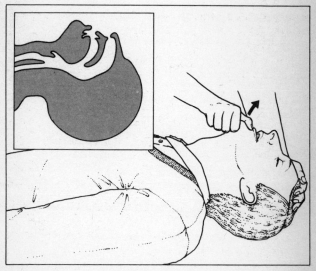

Chin lift.

Teaching hints

Demonstrate the head tilt and chin lift methods of opening the airway on the head section model supplied with your manikin. Overhead projector overlay transparencies are a good means of illustrating the structures involved to a large class. Alternatively the AMBU Intubation Trainer which has a cross-sectional cut-away is an excellent, though expensive, model for demonstration. Get your students to practise head tilt and chin lift on one another.

Some common questions

Q Will it help to put a pillow under the victim's head?
A No. Any object used to position the head will only make the obstruction worse. Never put anything under the head of an unconscious casualty. However, in an infant a pad of some sort placed between the shoulder blades may be helpful in keeping the head tipped back.

Q Is it possible to tilt the head too far?
A Yes – in certain circumstances.

1 When you suspect a neck injury: take great care not to tilt the head back too far – it might cause damage to the spinal cord.
2 In infants: because the neck is short and chubby, over-extending the neck may cause the relatively soft windpipe to kink.
3 In elderly patients: the main blood supply to the brain passes through the neck and some arteries go through tunnels in the neck bones. In old people wear and tear in the neck may have made these channels narrower than usual, and because they also tend to have hardened arteries over-extending the neck can cause kinking in these blood vessels.

Checking for breathing

Having opened the airway by tilting the head back and lifting the chin forward the rescuer should next check to see if the casualty is breathing. Look, listen and feel for breathing.

● Look – at the casualty's chest to see that it is rising and falling.
● Listen – for the breath sounds.
● Feel – for the warm air escaping from the casualty's mouth and nose.

(Some people teach their classes to feel for movements of the rib cage. This is sometimes useful though a little unnecessary.)

Some common questions

Q Sometimes on films we see actors checking for breathing with a mirror held against the victim's mouth – the mirror steams up which shows he's breathing. Is this method any good?

A Yes – but how many people, men in particular, carry a mirror everywhere they go? 'Look, listen and feel' needs eyes, ears and hands only.

In many cases opening the airway will have been enough to allow breathing to restart even though the casualty may still be unconscious. If so, the rescuer should turn him into the recovery position and stay with him until help arrives. If not rescuers should check that the airway is not still blocked by inclining the head towards one side and sweeping the hooked index finger quickly around the inside of the mouth to pull out any obvious obstruction.

THE RECOVERY POSITION

Some people would claim that of all the resuscitation procedures, the recovery position is the single most valuable action in saving lives, yet its use is frequently overlooked. You could perhaps begin this part of the session by explaining that the problems associated with an unconscious casualty are not restricted to the tongue going floppy and blocking the throat. Several other complications may develop as well: the protective reflexes which stop particles from slipping from the mouth into the lungs may be out of action; coughing may be depressed; the risk of vomiting is increased; digestive juices accumulate in the throat and stomach because the normal removal mechanisms have failed; the emptying of the stomach is delayed and the muscles guarding the entrance to the stomach relax. This means there is an increased risk of the stomach contents being regurgitated and these may spill over into the lungs. This is particularly likely to happen if the casualty is left lying on his back. Turning the casualty onto his side will:

● reduce the likelihood of the tongue falling back against the throat;
● allow any fluid or vomit to drain out of the mouth rather than spill into the lungs.

There are many different ways to turn someone onto her side and several different final positions in which she may be nursed. You will probably have heard different descriptive terms being used for the same manoeuvre: the recovery position; the three-quarter prone position; the semi-prone position; the lateral position; the coma position; the unconscious position; the side stable position, and so on.

Research from Australia suggests that turning the

victim into a position with the lower arm stretched out gives the best position for keeping the airway open and allows the most efficient use of the breathing muscles. The traditional teaching in the United Kingdom has recommended turning the casualty towards the rescuer with the lower arm underneath the victim and then pulling it out behind. We do not think that it really matters which position you choose to follow and teach, providing that you use and teach it well and that it meets the following criteria:

1   The procedure should minimise the movement of the casualty.
2   The casualty's head, neck and trunk should be kept in a straight line.
3   The position should allow gravity draining of liquid from the casualty's mouth.
4   The position should be stable, ie the casualty should not be able to fall over or topple into any other position. (Recommendations from the International League of Red Cross and Red Crescent Societies.)

Here we described two methods for turning the casualty onto her side. The first technique is that described in the *First Aid Manual* and demonstrated in the BBC TV *Save A Life* programme – you may prefer to follow this during the campaign. The second method is the Australian method mentioned above. You may have learnt another method and have a personal preference for it. The most important thing is to learn one method – whichever you feel confident to practise and teach – and use this method exclusively. Be able to explain and justify its features. Using more than one technique confuses and overwhelms the students.

Method I
This is the accepted method in the UK. It is easy to teach and to learn. It also has an advantage that it can be used in a relatively confined space, and the body and, in particular, the head of the victim can be properly

25

supported by the rescuer. To turn the unconscious casualty lying on her back onto her side:

1　Kneel beside her level with her chest. Tilt her head back and lift the chin upwards so that you keep her airway open.

2　Place the arm nearest you by the casualty's side then slide her hand palm upwards underneath her buttock. Bring her other arm up, bend it and lay it across the chest. Cross her further ankle over her nearer ankle.

3　Support the casualty's head with one hand. Use the other to grasp the clothes at the hip furthest away from you. Now gently roll the casualty towards you until she is resting against your knees.

4　Readjust her head to make sure her airway is still open.

5　Bend the casualty's uppermost arm and then the uppermost leg. This prevents the casualty rolling on to her face.

6　Ease out her other arm and leave it lying parallel to her back. This prevents her rolling back.

Method II

A criticism frequently levelled at the 'standard' recovery position is that the casualty's weight causes the body to topple over into the three-quarter prone position whereby the ribs become squashed and breathing is impaired. The position of the arms and legs in Method II keeps the chest off the ground and ensures efficient use of the breathing muscles. It has proved popular in Australia for near-drowning cases where it has been named the 'side stable' position. It is likely to become the standard method for the future.

To turn the unconscious casualty lying on his back onto his left side:

1　Stretch out the casualty's left arm horizontally until it is 90° to his body. Bring the casualty's right arm across his chest.

2 Bend the right knee to bring the thigh up at right angles to the hip keeping the left leg straight.

3 Now kneel at the casualty's right side and roll him towards the left by grasping his clothing firmly at the hip and shoulder. Ensure that you turn the casualty smoothly keeping the spine in its natural line. A second rescuer, if available, could support the head and keep the airway open.

4 Now that the victim is on his left side place his right arm across the left arm at the elbow. If the casualty has very broad shoulders it may be useful to put his left hand under his head so that it does not flop sideways onto the floor. Adjust the head to give the best position.

5 Open the airway. The face should be turned slightly downwards allowing drainage of saliva and vomit. Before leaving the casualty to get help make sure that his airway is clear and unimpeded and that he is still breathing.

Teaching hints

You will need a fairly large floor area and a blanket or ground sheet spread out. Each member of your group should have a chance to be both casualty and rescuer. Emphasise that the aim is to get the casualty into a position which is both safe *and* comfortable. It's only when you have been laid in the recovery position with a bulky set of keys in your back pocket that you appreciate exactly what this means. Demonstrate the recovery position using the smallest member of the class to turn the largest member. This shows how easy it is even for the physically disadvantaged to be aided by the pull of gravity and the patient's weight. Start by teaching the manoeuvre to turn the casualty onto one side only, say, the left side. When your students have gained confidence, try testing their application of knowledge by asking them to turn the casualty the other way – onto the right side. At the end of the class encourage your students to practise the recovery position at home on other members of the family or friends.

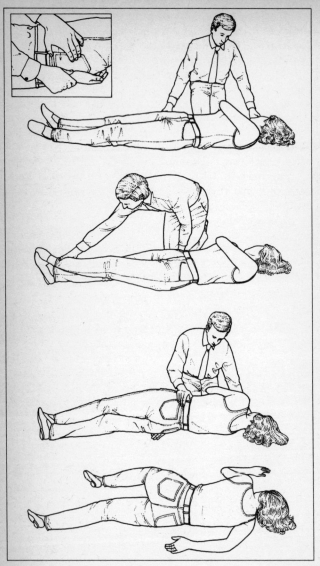

Recovery position: Method 1.

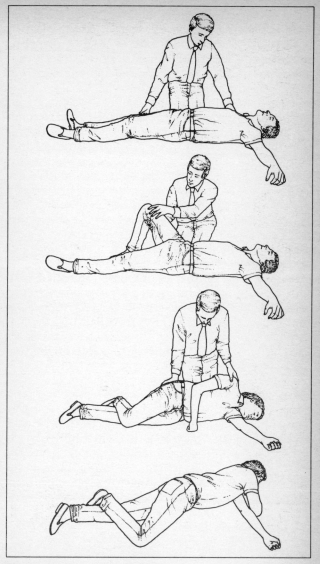

Recovery position: Method II.

Neck or spinal injuries

Students should be advised when using the recovery position to take particular care in cases of suspected spinal injury; for example, from road traffic accidents, falls from ladders or down stairs, horseriding accidents, rugby scrum mishaps, dives into shallow water. You will need to emphasise that, although damage may occur, students must not be discouraged from attempting first aid. It may help to explain how the vertebrae sit naturally one on top of the other supported by thick muscle. This allows the small joints at each side of the spine to move rather than the individual bones. Even with the relaxed muscles of an unconscious casualty these bones fit naturally together, and despite individual neck bones being broken this normal pattern may still be retained. Nevertheless if the neck bones are badly damaged the casualty must obviously be handled very carefully. Turning the head from side to side or extending it too far may cause injured spinal bones to slide on each other cutting or compressing the spinal cord. The best way to ensure that the bones remain in the normal position is to keep the spine as straight as possible (moving the casualty – if it is really necessary – in such a way as to keep this line) and to extend (but not over-extend) the neck gently when the person is put into the recovery position.

One of the common faults in handling cases of spinal injury is to turn the casualty too far so that she is, in fact, almost lying on her stomach. This can be dangerous when the nerves to the chest muscles are paralysed for the chest becomes immobilised and breathing may be restricted. To avoid turning the casualty too far a rescuer may have to support her body with a cushion, pillow or rolled blanket.

Some common questions

Q What if the casualty is not lying on his back?

A If the casualty is lying in a position that maintains his airway it is unnecessary to alter that position. If he

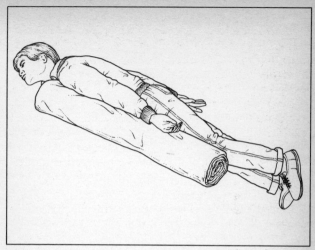

Recovery position for suspected spinal injuries.

is lying face downwards it is only necessary to make sure his airway is clear (but note the comments about spinal injuries opposite). In other positions the aim should be the same – to move the casualty as little as possible whilst establishing a clear airway with a slight downward tilt.

Q Once I've turned the casualty onto his side is it safe to leave him?
A Yes, this is the stage at which you can go and search for help. But before you leave the casualty, do re-check the airway, breathing and pulse as it is fairly common for an unconscious casualty's condition to get worse. Try not to leave the unconscious casualty unattended any longer than is absolutely necessary.

B BREATHING

Mouth-to-mouth breathing

'Expired air resuscitation' is probably the oldest form
of artificial ventilation described. The reference to
mouth-to-mouth rescue breathing in the Old Testa-
ment of the Bible is well known. This was when Elisha
the prophet revived the son of the Shunammite woman.

'. . . And he went up and lay upon the child and put his
mouth upon his mouth and his eyes upon his eyes and his
his hands his hands, and he stretched forth himself upon the
child and the flesh of the child waxed warm. . . .' Kings II 4.

Similar mention is made in ancient Egyptian and
Hebrew texts. It is also understood that midwives in
the twelfth century used expired air methods in re-
suscitating infants at birth.

There is a fascinating account of mouth-to-mouth
breathing in a paper given to the Royal Society in 1745
when William Tossach, a surgeon from Alloa in Perth-
shire, attended a miner in respiratory arrest (probably
from methane intoxication) after a colliery disaster.

'The colour of the skin of his body was natural, except where
it was covered with coal dust; his eyes were staring open,
and his mouth was gaping wide; his skin was cold; there was
not the least pulse in either the heart or arteries, and not the
least breathing could be observed: so that he was in all
appearances dead.

Tossach then described how he had to pinch the nostrils
in order to get a tight fit and how an apparently normal
recovery took place.

'I applied my mouth close to his and blowed my breath as
strong as I could; but having neglected to stop his nostrils,
all the air came out at them: wherefore, taking hold of them
with one hand, and holding my other on his breast at the

32

left pap, I blew again my breath as strong as I could, raising his chest fully with it; and immediately I felt six or seven very quick beats of the heart; his thorax continued to play, and the pulse was felt soon after in the arteries. . . . After about an hour he began to yawn, and to move his eye-lids, hands, and feet. . . . In an hour more he came pretty well to his senses and could take drink; but knew nothing of all that had happened . . . Within four hours he walked home, and in as many days returned to his work.'

The explanation for the success of mouth-to-mouth breathing is that our exhaled air contains 16% oxygen – more than enough to spare for those who are short. This fact was not realised by scientists like Lavoisier and Priestly – the 'discoverers' of oxygen – who condemned the technique as being unnatural. From the time of the foundation of the (Royal) Humane Society for the Recovery of Persons Apparently Drowned by Dr William Hawes in 1774 to the middle of this century, there were hundreds of methods of artificial resuscitation described. These included postural manoeuvres and manual methods where pressure on the chest and lifting of the arms aimed to shift air in and out of the lungs.

In the 1950s Dr James Elam and Dr Peter Safar at the Baltimore City Hospital in the USA and Professor Brophy in Brisbane, Australia, carried out tests to compare the effectiveness of the various manual methods with the mouth-to-mouth breathing technique. Their results clearly showed that the latter method was far superior. Neither the Holger Neilsen nor the Silvester methods (which were the most popular of the manual ones) produced enough movements of air to support life. For any method of ventilation to work the airway must be open – with the manual methods the airway is largely ignored. In 1958 Professor Safar even showed in an experiment using anaesthetised medical students with clear airways supported by tracheal tubes, that blood oxygen levels actually fell during the use of these methods. All that was happening was that the same air was being moved up and down the airway. So these methods are of no benefit to the casualty – they are not 'alternative' methods and should not be taught to people.

Some common questions

Q What if the patient has severe face and nose injuries?
A It is still inappropriate to use a method which does not work. Attempt to establish an airway, perhaps covering the injury with a clean handkerchief, or gently lift the broken jaw forwards to clear the airway, and then attempt to give mouth-to-mouth ventilation. There are even instances on record where heroic first aiders have attempted to make a hole in the windpipe with a pen knife to allow in air below an obstruction. This rare act is justified if no other help is available, for the patient would definitely die if left without oxygen.

Q Can the lungs be damaged by over-blowing?
A In adults a rescuer will not damage the victim's lungs through overblowing – after all the air came from his or her own lungs which had to expand to contain it! When practising on a manikin your students should be able to feel the resistance at the end of an inflation. Explain that they will feel this resistance after an adequate inflation in any casualty, even when giving small breaths in children. Students will feel more confident if they realise that they are not going to cause damage.

Four rapid full breaths

The four initial 'staircase' breaths recommended are intended to act as a trigger to the patient's own breathing:

● by stimulating the stretch receptors in the lungs (the reflex response is often enough to re-start breathing);
● by letting the additional effect of the rescuer's carbon dioxide stimulate the breathing centre in the victim's brain.

Recent research in the United States has suggested that giving breath too fast and at too great a pressure does not improve oxygen supply but distends the stomach. This is most likely in two-man CPR (pp. 44–45) when there is very little time in which to interpose a breath after every fifth chest compression. However, it also affects one-man CPR at the beginning of mouth-to-mouth breathing in the 'four quick breaths' sequence. The evidence was so impressive that the American Heart Association have decided to replace four initial breaths with two slower ones in their recommendations for emergency resuscitation. The *Save A Life* Campaign will continue to teach the four breaths manoeuvre since most instructors are used to this technique and it provides satisfactory results. Frequent changes of technique cause anxiety and should be discouraged. Note, however, the subtle change in the text – 'four rapid *full* breaths', and these are better *not* stepped but should allow the chest to fall between breaths. It is recommended that the four breaths are spread over 10–15 seconds.

Teaching hints
If a student fails to inflate the lungs of the training manikin, check whether:

1 the head is tilted fully back;
2 the nose is properly pinched off;
3 there is a tight seal around the lips.

Lack of success is invariably due to one of these factors.

Variations
Expired air resuscitation is a technique not merely restricted to mouth-to-mouth breathing. *Mouth-to-nose* breathing is equally effective, especially in drowning emergencies, but one problem with this technique is that if there is blockage of the nostrils (eg because of nasal polyps) then exhalation of the air blown in may be obstructed. For this reason we recommend that in mouth-to-nose breathing the casualty's mouth be

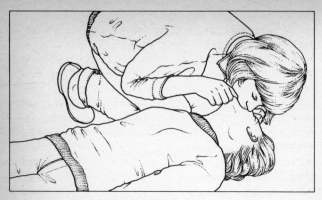

1 Is the head tilted fully back?
2 Is the nose properly pinched off?
3 Is there a good seal around the lips?

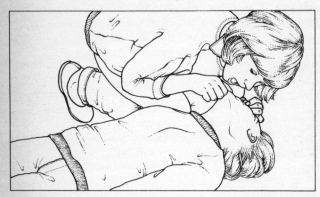

4 Is the chest rising and falling?

opened by the rescuer to allow the release of air. *Mouth-to-stoma* breathing should be used when the victim has a tracheostomy. This is an artificial hole made in the windpipe for medical reasons. In some people, eg those who have had surgery for cancer of the larynx, this is permanent and is the main entrance to the airway. In small children and babies an adult rescuer's mouth easily covers both mouth and nose (see p. 70).

Some common questions

Q What is the risk of catching a serious disease like AIDS from mouth-to-mouth resuscitation?

A This particular question is one of the commonest asked by students at present. It is difficult to give a reasonable answer without having a little bit of background knowledge; for this reason an appendix 'Some notes on AIDS' appears at the back of this book. However, you can tell your class that the chance of getting AIDS from rescue breathing is calculated to be less than one in a million. (Compare this with the one in 5000 chance of dying in a car accident.) Although mouth-to-mouth resuscitation has been used on thousands of occasions – and many lives undoubtedly saved as a result – no transmission of any lethal germ, including AIDS and hepatitis, has been reported. What is more, although over 40 000 000 Americans have learned CPR using training manikins, and perhaps as many as 150 000 000 persons worldwide, 'to our knowledge the use of CPR manikins has never been documented as being responsible for an outbreak or even an isolated case of bacterial, fungal or virus disease' (Center for Disease Control, Atlanta, Georgia, 1983). Further declaration of the safety of mouth-to-mouth breathing is given in a statement in the current (American) Standards and Guidelines on Cardiopulmonary Resuscitation and Emergency Cardiac Care (see p. 144 for more statistics on this subject).

No-one can state categorically that there is no risk of catching *any* type of germ attached to resuscitation – the transmission of cold sores by mouth-to-mouth contact probably occurs fairly frequently and there will be cases (eg the gutter drunk) where even the least squeamish will think twice before performing expired air resuscitation. Luckily, however, our students at CPR classes are self-selected. Those with real fears of passing on or getting an infection will probably not attend the classes anyway.

Q What are your views about the use of resuscitation aids?

A We assume you are referring to devices such as the Brooke or other Airway, with or without a one way valve; and the various types of pocket mask and more sophisticated devices such as the bag-valve-mask unit. Generally the use of these devices by members of the public is to be discouraged because of the real chance that the device will not be available when the need for resuscitation arises. Basic life support manoeuvres use the hands and breath alone – these are always available. But if the ownership of resuscitation devices (which might be kept, for example, in the glove compartment of a car) means that your students would feel happier about giving resuscitation to a stranger, then we should not criticise people for carrying them. And in this case it is essential that proper training in their use is given. This technically becomes part of the remit of Advanced Life Support Classes.

C CIRCULATION

Is there a pulse?
One of the biggest mistakes in the performance of
resuscitation is banging on the victim's chest without
checking to see whether the heart has stopped beating,
ie whether there is a pulse. It is essential, as an instructor, that you make it absolutely clear that chest compressions must only be used to support the circulation
when the pulse is absent – instil into your class the
fundamental importance of the pulse check.

Make it clear too that it's no use checking the pulse
at the wrist. In someone whose circulation is impaired
because of heart disease or shock, the radial (wrist)
pulse is unreliable. Listening to the chest itself is of no
use either, even with a stethoscope, and you will have
difficulty feeling for the heart beat in the chest. So one
of the more central major pulses should be checked,
and the choice lies between the femoral pulse in the
groin and the carotid pulse in the neck. For obvious
reasons, exposure of the groin in public is to be avoided!
Therefore the carotid pulse is preferred.

The main advantage of the neck pulse is that it
reflects, most accurately, the presence of blood flow to
the head and brain. It is useful therefore not merely as
the way of checking whether a circulation is present or
absent, but also as a means of gauging the effectiveness
of chest compressions. Spend some time with your
class going over the technique of feeling for the carotid
pulse. Explain the landmarks: the larynx (voice box),
and its Adams Apple; the strap muscle (the sterno-
mastoid) running obliquely across the neck; and the
groove between these structures containing the pulse.
Explain that in an elderly person or someone with loose
skin in the neck, you may have to press fairly deeply
backwards in order to locate this point. Get your

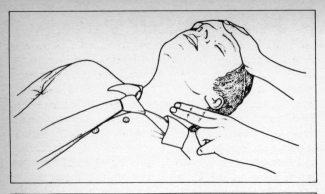

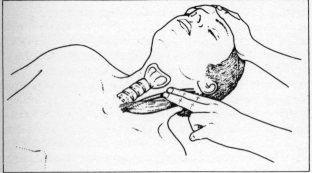

Feeling for the carotid pulse.

students to practise feeling for the pulse on themselves and on one another. Let them see the difference in position and strength of the pulse between the subject sitting up and lying down.

Do be absolutely certain that the heart has stopped. People who appear to be in cardiac arrest might just have a very slow pulse (bradycardia), for example, from fainting; others may have missed a beat because of irregularities in the heart's action. Having located the position of the pulse, rescuers should count slowly up to five. If no pulse is felt during this time they can assume that the heart beat is absent and they should begin chest compressions.

Chest compression

The techniques of closed chest cardiac compression came into common use as recently as 1960 (just over 26 years ago) as a result of investigations carried out by Drs Kouwenhoven, Knickerbocker and Jude from the Johns Hopkins Hospital in Baltimore. Whilst undertaking laboratory experiments on defibrillation of the heart, they noticed that by rhythmically pressing down upon the animal's chest so as to compress the area in between its breastbone and spine they could achieve an adequate pressure of blood (approximately 80 mm of mercury) in the blood vessels to the brain. It has since been shown that over a third of the normal circulation (cardiac output) can be obtained by properly performed chest compressions and this is sufficient to keep the brain supplied with oxygen.

How this actually works has been the subject of considerable debate with two different schools of thought emerging. The long-held belief (and the easiest concept to put across to lay people) is the Heart Pump Theory. This is that 'pressure on the sternum compresses the heart between it and the spine, forcing out blood'. Recent studies indicate that this is not entirely true. According to the Chest Pump Theory, most of the movement of blood occurs because of the sucking-in action of the chest cage when compression is released with the heart being nothing more than a passive conducting tube. Such experimental work over the years has led to the most efficient and most easily taught methods of chest compression being evolved. The 'standard' technique described here takes all the various scientific considerations into account.

The *First Aid Manual* describes what has been nicknamed as the 'halving method' of identifying the lower half of the breastbone. The breastbone is bisected by placing the thumbs midway between the landmarks – the notch at the top and the junction with the ribs at the bottom. We prefer the 'two fingers method'. A right-handed person places two fingers of his right hand

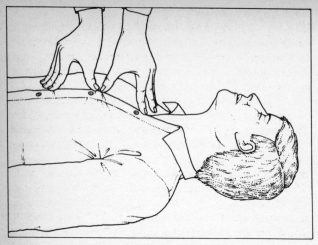

Finding the midpoint of the lower half of the sternum – the 'halving technique'.

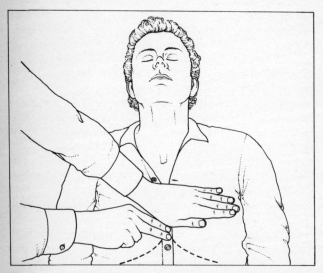

Finding the midpoint of the lower half of the sternum – the 'two fingers technique'.

immediately above the base of the breastbone (the xiphisternum or the xiphoid) and the base of his left hand immediately above this point. This method is quick to perform and allows for accurate re-positioning of the hands between ventilations and compressions.

You should encourage your students to aim for as near perfect chest compressions as possible. The compressions should be regular and smooth, and the downstroke should take slightly longer than the release. The hands should never be out of contact with the chest wall.

● Properly performed chest compressions are better for the victim – they allow for the most efficient pumping of the blood.

● Properly performed chest compressions are better for the rescuer – they are less tiring and do not impose a strain or fatigue on the rescuer's arms.

● Improperly performed chest compressions may cause damage to the victim including broken ribs and lung injury.

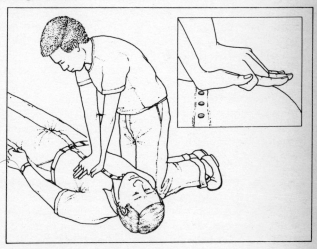

Are the elbows straight?
Are the fingers clear of the chest?

Teaching hints
There are several common pitfalls to watch out for:

1 The *bouncing technique* with both elbows. Sharp, often too rapid jabs at the patient's chest are very tiring for the operator and do not allow the casualty's heart to re-fill with blood adequately between jabs. Use of the term 'cardiac massage' should be discouraged as this does tend to suggest bouncing compressions. The bouncing technique can be avoided by ensuring that the elbows are kept straight and by counting '1 – and, 2 – and', etc. On the count of the number you press down, on the count of the word 'and' you release.

2 The *rocking chair technique.* Rocking to and fro from the waist is inefficient, the squeezing action on the heart is poor and the method is likely to break ribs. The action should be a downwards compression with arms straight from the shoulders, positioned vertically above the casualty's heart.

3 The *crossed or splayed hands technique.* This spreads the impact of the compressions on to the chest cage and is likely to lead to broken ribs. Only the heel of the hand should make contact with the sternum – this can be achieved by locking the fingers together and pulling them upwards off the chest.

4 *Wrong hand position.* There is a tendency for a rescuer to press too low down (over the xiphoid) or drift across to the patient's left. Bad hand positions can lead to internal injury of the abdominal organs or lungs. Such problems can be avoided by re-checking the hand position with each change from ventilation to compression.

Remember that both mouth-to-mouth respiration *and* external chest compression are needed in a cardiac arrest. The exact technique will depend on whether the rescuer is on his own or if there is another person to help. If he is on his own, he should alternate 15 compressions (at the rate of about 80 per minute) with two breaths. Resuscitation where two rescuers are involved

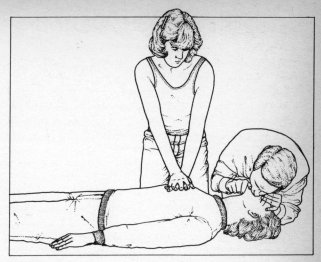

Where there are two rescuers, a rate of 5 compressions to 1 breath should be aimed for.

cannot be adequately taught in a single session training class. The additional manoeuvres and different ratios only serve to confuse people who have mostly come to training classes in order to prepare themselves for the emergency they may face on their own – say, in their own home. The experience of the Seattle researchers is that when two-rescuer resuscitation is performed one of the rescuers almost always turns out to be a health care professional. CPR instructors, of course, must be totally familiar with one-rescuer and two-rescuer resuscitation. Be prepared to demonstrate (but not to try and teach) two-rescuer resuscitation to interested members of your group if time permits.

If there are two rescuers present one should carry out external chest compression uninterrupted at a rate of about 60 per minute whilst the other should provide one breath every fifth compression. The rescuer performing mouth-to-mouth resuscitation should check every three minutes for the return of the carotid pulse.

Successful resuscitation may be gauged by:

- the return of the carotid pulse
- a return to normal colour of the face and lips
- the appearance of the pupils. In cardiac arrest with reduced blood flow to the brain the pupils of the eyes will dilate (get wider). This is not always a reliable sign and so should not be used to diagnose cardiac arrest. However, return of the pupil size to normal may be a good indicator that brain resuscitation has been successful – pupils which remain wide and unreactive usually indicate that revival is unlikely.

Some common questions

Q Why give both mouth-to-mouth breathing and chest compressions?

A Rescue breathing is needed to get oxygen into the blood stream. Chest compressions are needed to pump the blood to the tissues of the body. Unless *both* the breathing and circulation are being supported oxygen cannot be transported to the vital parts of the body.

Q 15:2. 5:1. 80 per minute. 60 per minute. Why do you recommend these specific ratios and rates?

A The answer is one of logic and practicality rather than being based on any strong scientific reasons. The average normal breathing rate for human beings is 12–15 breaths per minute and the average heart rate 60–80 per minute. Resuscitation would be performed optimally at these rates. This can be achieved in two-rescuer CPR since 60 compressions per minute is the normal heart rate, and every five seconds a breath is given, ie 12 breaths per minute – again the normal rate. In one-rescuer CPR time is lost with each change from compression to ventilation, so a rate of 5:1 becomes technically unachievable. However, by administering two full breaths the lungs become saturated with oxygen which does not start to become used up until a further three cycles, ie 15 compressions, have taken place. The chest will need compressing a little faster than one per second, ie 80 times per minute, to compensate for the compressions that are not given while the ventilation is being performed.

Q Do you no longer recommend the chest thump?

A The 'precordial' or chest thump was at one time recommended as a CPR technique in cardiac arrest because:

● it may stimulate the heart's own pacemaker when the heart has missed a beat;

● it may halt runs of life-threatening rhythm abnormalities, eg ventricular fibrillation.

Because it can occasionally bring on ventricular fibrillation and, in the absence of a defibrillator, this may have a fatal outcome, use of the precordial thump has only been recommended for witnessed arrests on monitored patients in hospital. Since confusion was arising over what constituted a witnessed arrest and since, in order to be performed properly, the precordial thump became yet another technique to have to be very carefully taught, it was decided to exclude it from the *Save A Life* curriculum. We are sure that it will continue to be used, in appropriate circumstances, in special care areas of hospitals.

BLEEDING

The ABC of resuscitation is only going to be successful if there is sufficient blood in the system. The red blood cells of the body carry oxygen to the tissues. This oxygen is used to burn up energy, and carbon dioxide, the waste product of this burning, is carried away by those circulating cells to the lungs. Here it is exchanged for more oxygen.

People who are bleeding very slowly (from ulcers in the stomach or bowel) can often manage to walk about with only half their normal ration of haemoglobin (the oxygen-carrying pigment in the red cells). Accident victims start to feel faint, develop rapid pulses and faster breathing after a much smaller drop than this.

So what types of injuries result in significant blood loss? Advise your students that superficial scratches and abrasions, even if they cover quite a large area, can usually be ignored because the small blood vessels of the skin itself are able to close up quite quickly after injury. Instead they should watch out for wounds, even apparently quite small ones, in larger deeper blood vessels. These are unable to close up because the blood rushes out too quickly for the normal clotting action to take place and if pressure is not applied promptly, the body's blood volume will fall to a dangerously low level.

Students often ask why blood clots at the site of a wound but stays liquid in our circulation. Briefly, the mechanism of clotting is that when blood escapes from blood vessels a substance called 'fibrin' is released which forms a fine mesh over the wound and triggers the release of clotting agents. The combination of fibrin and clotted blood seals the wound and blocks the escape of more blood. Our aim as rescuers is to slow down the flow of blood from an injury so that this clotting process can occur. This can be done by several means:

1 Making it difficult for blood to escape by applying local pressure – a firm pad or even fingers held over the wound;

2 Closing the wound if it has gaping edges – bringing the sides of a straight cut together by pushing on either side;

3 Where possible, lifting up the damaged part, eg an arm or leg, to increase the height up to which the heart needs to pump blood and so slow down the flow.

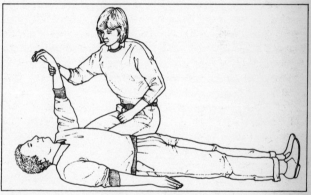

Apply pressure over the wound and if possible elevate the limb.

If applying a pad does not stop the bleeding, rescuers should not try to remove it as it will already be involved in the clotting process. They should put a further firm dressing on top.

Dressings should be firm enough to stop bleeding but not tight enough to stop circulation reaching beyond the wound. Tell your students to make sure fingers and toes still go white when pressed with a finger and that the colour returns when they take it off. In the rare cases of part of an arm or leg being cut or torn off completely, pressure must be as tight as possible to stop blood escaping from torn arteries.

Some common questions
Q Is it true that we no longer use tourniquets and pressure points?
A Most bleeding can be controlled by firm local pressure and, if a limb is bleeding, by lifting it above the level of the heart. In very rare circumstances, when a deep artery is cut, such as in cases of amputation, it may be that you will need to find the point where the artery is nearer the surface and crosses over a bone so that it can be compressed more easily. This area is called a pressure point and firm pressure should be applied. However, every 10 minutes the pressure should be released, otherwise the tissues beyond that point will die through lack of oxygen. In the case of a complete amputation, this pressure can be permanent because there is no tissue to save and you need to conserve as much blood as possible in the circulation.

CHOKING

Most of us have had personal experience of some form of 'choking' but when the airway is completely obstructed then choking becomes an alarming and potentially fatal emergency. The obstruction is usually a foreign body – food in adults, beads, marbles, toys etc. in children – which has become lodged in the windpipe. If foreign bodies completely obstruct the air passages in the larynx, the victim will be unable to speak or breathe and will instinctively clutch at his throat. He will become pale, then progress to unconsciousness. Unfortunately sometimes when this happens the victim may have time to escape from the dining table to the bathroom hoping to make himself sick. Often this departure goes un-noticed. Your class is a good opportunity to stress the danger of this behaviour. Encourage people to draw attention to themselves if they think they are choking, however self-conscious they may feel.

Explain briefly to your class the anatomy of the air passages. The upper airway branches into two large tubes – the main bronchi, and then a series of smaller tubes. All these contain air. It follows that if you can get all this air pushing upwards at great pressure there is a good chance of moving the obstruction. The best way of obtaining a high pressure is for all the victim's muscles to be used in a co-ordinated effort – the small muscles in between the ribs, the muscles of the neck and chest wall, and the diaphragm. This occurs when the person coughs. Further assistance can be obtained from gravity.

There is no time to waste. Tell your students to gain the victim's confidence by taking hold of his shoulders, looking him in the eyes and speaking calmly and firmly. They should first confirm that his airway is completely blocked by asking if he can speak. If he cannot, they should lean him over a chair and tell him to cough as hard as he can. You should, of course, also point out that this is how students should deal with choking if they themselves are ever victims in such a situation. (If the person can speak but is sure there is something lodged in his windpipe, still encourage him to cough with his head down. If despite this he becomes unconscious, it is particularly worth trying mouth-to-mouth breathing as the fact that he could speak means there may still be a partial airway open.)

Should these measures fail, the air behind the object can be compressed by firm back blows – four firm blows between the shoulder blades while the casualty is leaning head down over the chair. If this also fails the casualty will be becoming short of oxygen and fall unconscious. The rescuer should place him on the floor and attempt to hook the foreign body out with his index finger. If there is still no obvious success, he should attempt to open the airway and give mouth-to-mouth breathing – the object may have moved into one of the bronchi allowing one lung to be inflated. Enough oxygen is available from one lung to restore consciousness and allow time to get the casualty to hospital. If no air enters the lungs (ie the chest does not rise) the rescuer should repeat back blows after rolling the casualty to his side, then again try finger sweeps and attempt mouth-to-mouth.

The American Heart Association recommends that abdominal thrusts (the 'Heimlich Manoeuvre') be used exclusively in cases of obstructed airway. We are not convinced by the evidence so far produced and suggest that this technique is only tried after back blows and finger sweeps have failed. The technique can be demonstrated on resuscitation models such as Resusci Anne but should not be demonstrated on your students because of the danger of damaging the gullet or even the liver.

The procedure is as follows. Stand behind the person concerned and encircle the waist with your arms.

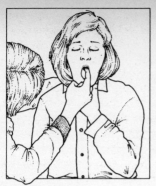

Finger sweeps

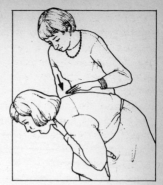

Back blows

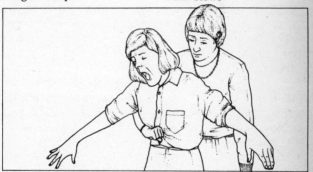

The abdominal thrust – form a fist with one hand

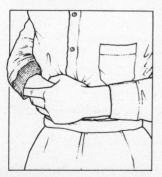

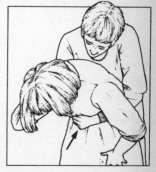

Grasp the fist and pull sharply upwards and inwards

With one hand make a fist and place it thumb side against the person's stomach between the navel and bottom of the breastbone (xiphisternum). Grasp the fist with your other hand and press into the person's stomach with a quick upward thrust so that the air remaining behind the obstruction is compressed with sufficient pressure to dislodge the object. It may be repeated up to six times if the first attempt is unsuccessful.

HEART ATTACKS

The concept of a heart attack is a difficult one to get across to students. There is often a misunderstanding of the principles and mixing up of terms. For example, the phrase 'heart attack' and 'cardiac arrest' are often confused.

The muscles of the heart receive their blood supply from the *coronary arteries* – so called because they spread around the heart like a crown (Latin – *corona*). If, for any reason, the blood supply from the coronary arteries is impaired then the amount of oxygen reaching the heart muscle is reduced and the heart does not function properly. Sometimes the blood flow in the coronary arteries is decreased because of narrowing of the arteries. When the heart's demand for oxygen increases, as during exercise for example, the blood flow through the narrow tubes is not able to meet the demand and a strain is put on the heart muscle leading to a state like cramp. This results in a condition known as *angina* where there is a stitch-like pain in the chest lasting for a minute or two but which disappears on resting.

Occasionally the obstruction in the coronary arteries comes on suddenly and completely; it may be because a blood clot forms – a *coronary thrombosis*. When this occurs a chunk of heart muscle supplied by the artery concerned actually dies and is no longer able to pump blood. The effect of this on the patient is to produce the symptoms and signs of heart attack. The medical name for a heart attack is *myocardial infarction* which, translated, means simply 'death of heart muscle'.

Heart attack is not necessarily the same as heart stoppage (cardiac arrest). Many people have made a full recovery from their heart attack because the pumping action of the heart muscle which dies is taken over by surrounding healthy muscle.

There are times though when the heart attack does result in cardiac arrest which, if not dealt with by resuscitation, leads to sudden death. This may be for two reasons:

● the amount of dead muscle is so great that no effective pumping action can take place.

● The heart attack interferes with the electrical rhythm of the heart resulting in ventricular fibrillation. This is when uncoordinated electrical activity in the heart muscle prevents the heart from pumping effectively. It can be reversed by using a machine known as a defibrillator, which shocks the muscle back into its proper rhythm.

The risk of sudden death occurring after the symptoms of a heart attack have been experienced drops off rapidly with time, but 75% of the cases of ventricular fibrillation occur within the first hour or so after the onset of symptoms. Hence the need for vigilance with a heart attack victim and the aim of an early and smooth transfer to medical aid.

Signs and symptoms

The signals which indicate a possible heart attack are:
● an uncomfortable feeling of pressure; gripping fullness of pain in the centre of the chest which may spread to arms, neck, throat, jaw and back.
● breathlessness
● severe giddiness or a feeling of weakness
● pale skin, heavy sweating, blue lips and finger tips.
A heart attack is often preceded by several days of feeling overwhelmingly tired and generally unwell. There may have been chest pain dismissed as 'indigestion'. The most severe chest pain rarely comes on abruptly. Typically it develops over several minutes.

The conditions of angina (the warning signs), myocardial infarction (the pathological state) and sudden death (from ventricular fibrillation), though obviously related, do not necessarily have to occur together. You can have angina without a heart attack, heart attack without angina or sudden death without either. But when the symptoms of angina or heart attack do occur they must be taken seriously and acted upon.

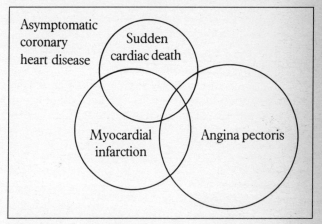

Heart disease – the inter-relation of myocardial infarction, angina and sudden death.

Some common questions
Q Can a heart attack be prevented?
A The straight answer to this question is yes. The amount of heart disease occurring in America has been reduced because of the effectiveness of awareness campaigns. One part of the American 'Heartsaver' Resuscitation Course is called 'Prudent Heart Living' and is dedicated to explaining the risk factors and preventive measures for heart attacks. Some risk factors, eg age, sex, genetic factors, etc., cannot be modified, but there are many that can. Cigarette smoking and high blood pressure are the two major risk factors. The risk of a heart attack is five times greater in smokers than in non-smokers. At your *Save A Life* class you must teach by example and actively discourage smoking – encourage your students to give up if they are heavy smokers.

People should also be encouraged to have their blood pressure checked regularly and treated if it starts to go too high. Other risk factors include stress, lack of exercise, being overweight and eating the wrong types of foods. A positive attitude to healthy living with the avoidance of a high-fat diet, regular exercise of a sustained nature such as swimming, cycling or jogging and the sort of life-style which seeks to avoid stressful circumstances goes a long way to reducing the risk of heart disease.

Q I know someone who has angina and he takes little tablets to put under his tongue. What are these for?
A These tablets, when absorbed through the mouth, reduce the work that the heart has to do. They are very effective in reducing the pain from angina. If someone with known angina experiences the signals of a heart attack it is useful to give him two of these tablets under the tongue. This may, to some extent, relieve the pain and reduce the feeling of unease. Chest pain which persists after taking two of these tablets is almost certainly from a heart attack and no time should be lost in following the treatment guide described.

Q Why don't you lie somebody flat when they have a heart attack?
A When somebody has had a heart attack their heart finds it difficult to pump blood around; it is also likely that fluid will accumulate in the lungs and make then less elastic. If you lie the patient flat the weight of the abdominal organs will squash the chest. If you sit the patient upright he will feel giddy because he has low blood pressure. The compromise is therefore to prop him up at a 45 degree angle; in this position he will find it easier to breathe.

DROWNING

Drowning means death by suffocation from immersion in water or other liquid, whether or not this liquid has entered the lungs.

Near-drowning is a more accurate term for cases where a person survives an immersion incident. Although initial resuscitation at the site of the accident may be successful, recovery is not complete at 24 hours and a stay in hospital is necessary.

Hypothermia means an abnormally low body temperature, usually resulting from accidental immersion in cold water or inadequate protection from a cold environment (especially when combined with high altitude, wind, moisture and physical exhaustion). It also arises from immobilisation and exposure to cold, especially in the unconscious, the elderly or seriously ill.

Drowning is the third commonest cause of accidental death (after road accidents and falls) and is surrounded by several myths which should be dispelled when discussing this topic with students. Rescuers are always concerned about the quantity of water in the lungs, but inhaling water does not in itself cause death. In experiments it has been shown that mammals can survive for several hours with their lungs filled with a salt solution, as long as it is saturated with oxygen. This is because the thin membrane lining the lungs allows gases to pass from the blood circulation into this water and vice versa. It has also been shown that there is no significant difference in the resuscitation techniques needed when patients drown in fresh, brackish or sea water, contrary to popular belief. Emphasise too that water does not need to be deep to be dangerous. Children can drown in even 1 or 2 inches of water and drowning accidents in the bath or shallow ponds are quite common. People should start resuscitation immediately. The only reason for pausing is if the airway appears to be obstructed. There is no need to bring a victim from the site of the drowning to land. Open the airway and proceed with mouth-to-mouth breathing in the water. Fortunately drowned victims are often fit young people with healthy hearts so there is a good chance of recovery as long as resuscitation occurs quickly.

Clearing the airway

Drowned victims usually float feet downwards and head upwards so it is fairly easy to tip the chin to produce a clear airway. Certain patients have such a dense body mass that their bodies are immersed almost completely with just their nose above the surface. On such an occasion a rescuer is much better to attempt to give mouth-to-nose resuscitation. If the airway appears to be obstructed the rescuer will find, unless he is an expert strong swimmer with a light victim, that it is difficult to do finger sweeps successfully. However, the obstruction may only be a small quantity of water above muscles in spasm and it is possible to 'blow past' this obstruction. Larger obstructions will need removal by finger sweeps so emphasise that it is important to keep trying this.

The danger of hypothermia

In British waters not only the victim but the rescuer can become very cold. Heat loss will be increased by making the effort to swim, particularly if towing another person, so if the rescuer has attracted attention and knows help is on its way it is easier to stay still with the victim giving mouth-to-mouth breaths rather than towing him to safety. People who can swim well in a pool forget how much energy is needed to swim in the colder rougher waters of the sea, for example. They because exhausted easily and they lose heat through their body surface.

Other dangers

People often ask why apparently strong fit swimmers drown, frequently when they are close to dry land. This is usually because their judgement or ability has been impaired – for example, by the cold, by alcohol, drugs or some form of injury.

Survival after immersion depends on several factors. Some people are capable of holding their breath for a very long time, and this is dependent upon their state of health and fitness immediately before the event and how long they had been exercising before getting into trouble. Victims who panic will use up extra heat (in addition to the usual amount lost from the body in water) because they use up so much energy by thrashing about. The body naturally attempts to make more breathing efforts in this situation, even after consciousness is lost, but, once unconscious, the muscles in the throat soon relax and water is then drawn into the lungs and stomach. If water has been drawn into the stomach earlier, this relaxation may also allow vomit to flow into the lungs as well. In a small number of drowning victims the muscles of the throat remain in spasm (laryngeal spasm) and the lungs are found to be dry at post mortem examination.

Secondary drowning

About 90% of drowning victims inhale some water into their lungs. Although, as we have said, inhaling water does not in itself necessarily cause death, the water does damage the membrane between the small blood vessels in the lungs and the airway where gases are exchanged. For this reason all immersion victims must be admitted to hospital as soon as possible to prevent what is known as 'secondary drowning'. This when fluid from the

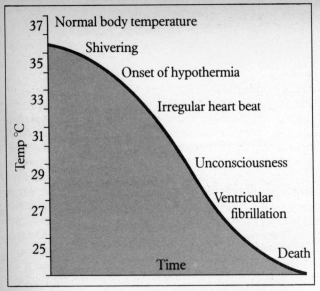

Hypothermia: the symptoms and signs at different body temperatures.

patient's own body fills the lungs via the damaged membrane some hours after the initial accident.

Recovery

In principle, most drowning victims will have got cold rapidly and not over several hours and they should be warmed up quickly too. They can either be immersed in a bath of warm water while awaiting the rescue services if their breathing has been restored, or be protected from the elements with blankets. Stress that the casualty is just as much at risk from becoming unconscious again as from 'secondary drowning' later, and a very close eye should be kept on him.

To sum up, the aim of resuscitation in drowning or near drowning victims is to restore the respiration and heart beat and to prevent further heat loss. Rescuers should never let a casualty be declared dead until he has been warmed up.

ROAD ACCIDENTS

Road accidents cause 39% of all accidental deaths in the UK and 78% of deaths in 15–19 age group. Although only 3% of miles travelled by motor vehicles are done by motor cycles, they are implicated in more than a quarter of fatal accidents. Most of us will be involved in an accident once in our lives. This is not just an area of anxiety for car users; pedestrians are frequently involved in accidents, particularly children and the elderly. All parents want to help their children by teaching them road drills and this part of the course will usually give rise to many questions. A lethargic class will often suddenly come to life at this point.

Here is a chance for the students to use all the skills they have learned. It is also a good opportunity for you to assess their grasp of the preceding sections. It will help if you paint a scenario and lead a discussion. For example, whilst walking the dog you hear a crash nearby and find two cars, each with four occupants, in a head-on collision (adapt the picture to suit your own environment). Discuss first the approach, then revise cardinal rules of emergency care:

1   Protect yourself
a)   Park safely (if in a car) well behind the accident site with your hazard lights flashing;

b)   Protect yourself. Do not run across motorway traffic to reach the other side;

c)   Be conspicuous – if you have no protective clothing at least try to wear something obvious. At night take off a dark coat if you have something more visible underneath – a white shirt or light-coloured dress;

d)   Look for other physical dangers. If a tanker is involved are there any Hazchem signs (note the details to pass on to the rescue services)? Is anyone smoking?

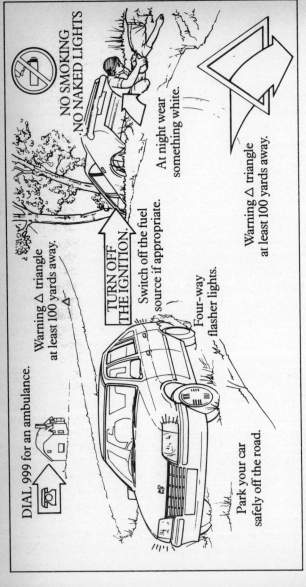

DIAL 999 for an ambulance.

Warning △ triangle at least 100 yards away.

NO SMOKING
NO NAKED LIGHTS

At night wear something white.

Warning △ triangle at least 100 yards away.

TURN OFF THE IGNITION.

Switch off the fuel source if appropriate.

Four-way flasher lights.

Park your car safely off the road.

Road accident: protecting the scene.

(Spilt petrol, though not easily ignited, is a fire hazard.) Is the engine still running in any involved vehicle? Switch it off and apply the handbrake if possible. Coaches and buses have an emergency fuel switch on the outside of the vehicle – ask members of the class to watch out for the various sites these are found on local buses. Can they describe where they have seen one?

2 Protect the accident site

This applies to rescuers and bystanders as well as the victims.

a) Park well behind the accident site and put on your car hazard lights;

b) Use a warning triangle;

c) Try to send someone to flag down traffic either side of the accident.

3 Assess the situation

Remember the cardinal rules of **A**irway, **B**reathing and **C**irculation. Ask students what they would do and in what order. Even in imaginary scenes you will find that one will correctly assess all the casualties quickly

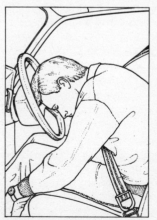 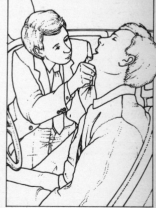

Opening the airway of a casualty in a car.

65

whereas another will spend the time with one victim only. Remind them that noisy patients are probably safer than quiet ones whose airways may be blocked. Beware a small quiet child unconscious on the rear seat or floor of the car, easily overlooked.

Here is a chance to highlight the importance of controlling major bleeding during resuscitation. Moving the casualty is not always necessary. Only if a victim is in obvious danger from fire or oncoming traffic should he be moved. Road traffic accident victims are often trapped in cars. Their airway and circulation can be controlled where they are. Spinal injuries should be presumed present until proved otherwise.

If the victim must be moved, rescuers should do so carefully keeping the head supported and the spine aligned. With an unconscious but breathing casualty they should remember to put him in the recovery position using the 'log roll' method.

4 Sending for help

Revise the '999' sequence. Rescuers should try to send someone responsible to call an ambulance but even a panicking casualty will calm down if given a task to do. There may be an unhurt passenger who can be sent. Discuss what information will be needed by the ambulance service and how to give clear directions. Is there a bystander who can wait at an obvious landmark to direct the ambulance driver? This person can also be given more updated details for the ambulance service so they know what equipment is required. On their ambulance radio they can call up further help or cancel it if it is no longer needed.

Students are often anxious about how to assume authority. Studies on crowds involved in major accidents show that victims respond to firm simple commands – authority comes from the rescuer's attitude, not his uniform or qualifications.

By taking charge calmly the rescuer will also quell

his own fears. The better his training and confidence, the higher his chance of success.

Many students will already have experienced road accidents. They may feel guilty about how they reacted. Constructive discussion will ease their guilt and prepare them for the next time. Help them accept that in a multiple casualty incident they have to do the best for all victims. This may mean leaving a pulseless, non-breathing victim to restore the airways of two others.

CHILDREN

Most parents, if they are honest, admit to feelings of concern and inadequacy at the thought of having to provide emergency treatment to a sick child, especially their own. This apprehension is often the principal motivating reason for adults enrolling in First Aid and Resuscitation classes. Your students' anxieties may be allayed by stressing that the *approach* to children is exactly the same as in adults and that the **ABC** principles learnt for adults can be applied equally to children. However, children are not just scaled-down grown ups – their bodily function is different and they suffer from different conditions to adults.

For example, heart attacks are fortunately very rare in children, and primary cardiac arrest is an extremely unusual event. However, children are still at risk from accidents in the home, on the roads, or in water, any of which may lead to airway and breathing problems. This difference must be stressed to your class. Most sick children are at risk mainly from a blocked airway or arrested breathing. Dashing in and pounding on the chest may not only cause considerable irreversible damage but is, most of the time, unnecessary: airway care and expired air resuscitation are usually the only techniques required. To reinforce this point, the *Save A Life* medical panel recommends that chest compressions in children are not included in the curriculum for a single-session class since there is not enough time to explain this technique properly and safely. Perhaps if there is sufficient local demand you might organise a special class (along the lines of the new American Red Cross 'Babysaver Course') to deal exclusively with emergency aid in infants and young children.

At the time of going to press the United Kingdom recommendations for resuscitation in infants and children are in their final draft form. For this reason our guidelines are based on current knowledge but, as with all medical matters, might require revision in the light of future research and experience.

Opening the airway

The airway in children is slightly shorter than in adults, the neck chubbier. Over-tilting of the head may cause kinking of the windpipe and so this should be avoided. A useful way of opening the airway of a baby lying on its back (eg in a cot) is to place one's hands under the shoulders and lift the shoulders up so that the head falls back naturally. Contact with the mattress (or whatever surface it is on) will prevent the head from falling back too far.

In the case of a feverish child with croup and marked breathing difficulty a rescuer should on no account put her finger down the child's throat to clear the airway – she may increase any inflammation present at the back of the throat in the dangerous and often unsuspected condition of *epiglottitis* and provoke a total airway obstruction.

Choking

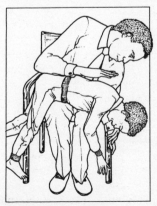

Back slaps for a child.

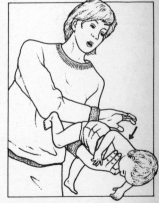

Back slaps for a baby.

Rescuers should treat a child in the same way as an adult. For a small child sit down and lay the child on his stomach over your knee, head down. Slap sharply between the shoulder blades 4 times. Use a little less force than you would use for an adult. For babies, lay the baby on his stomach along your arm, head down. Slap smartly but lightly between the shoulder blades.

Breathing

Expired air resuscitation in infants and children should be given by the *mouth to mouth and nose* method. Seal the child's mouth and nose with your mouth and blow gently into the lungs until the chest rises. Breathe at the rate of twenty breaths per minute (ever three seconds). Since you can breathe for a baby with him in your arms, ie you are not restricted to one place as you may be with an adult, carry the baby with you to a telephone giving breaths as you go.

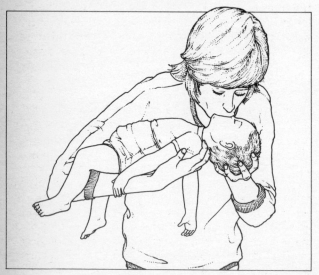

Covering the mouth and nose in a baby.

The pulse

This is best felt on the inside of the arm close to the armpit along the imaginary seam of a jacket sleeve. The pulse in children is proportionately faster than in an adult. .

Cardiac resuscitation in children

This is rarely necessary and can be dangerous if inexpertly performed. It is not included in the curriculum of the *Save A Life* class.

In children external chest compressions are performed with *one hand* at the rate of 80 compressions per minute. In babies use the *fingertips* and compress at the faster rate of about 100 per minute.

As instructors you will find yourself faced with lots of questions posed by anxious parents – questions which you may feel unable to answer. Do not fudge the answer. If you don't know, say so and suggest that the questioner seeks the specific advice of his or her family doctor. It is impossible to cover all emergency situations in children here, but we have included some short notes on three particularly worrying conditions.

Fits (convulsions)

Convulsions may occur in a child who has epilepsy or, more frequently, a high temperature (febrile convulsion). The child may look pale and ill, and start fitting in spasmodic jerks; the breathing may become noisy or difficult, perhaps with foaming at the mouth, and the child may lose control of bladder and bowel. The child may then lie still. During the fit a bystander should not move the child nor try to hold him down, nor put anything in his mouth. It is *after* the fit that the risk is greatest. He should then protect the airway by turning the child into the recovery position, then seek medical help. A prolonged fit or a second fit occurring within a quarter of an hour should be dealt with in hospital.

Asthma

Asthma is an alarming and potentially dangerous condition caused by obstruction of the lower airways, ie in the lungs themselves. Breathing is difficult and the sufferer becomes exhausted. A bystander should try to reassure and calm the victim and get him to sit or lean forward, supported, where there is a good supply of air. A child who suffers long term from asthma will probably have some medicine in the form of an aerosol inhaler – he should be helped to use it. Bystanders should be prepared to seek medical aid and give mouth-to-mouth breathing if breathing stops in a prolonged attack.

Cot death

This is a devastating experience for any parent. The sight of a baby, apparently lifeless in his cot, invokes all sorts of panic and guilt feelings – feelings which actually have no justification. Talk your students through such a situation. Tell them to try not to panic but to apply the approach to emergency aid and resuscitation that they have been taught. They should also seek help to get the baby to hospital. Even if the outcome is as they feared they will then at least know that everything that could have been done was done, and the medical and nursing staff will be able to offer the necessary help and support to face the sadness and sudden sense of loss.

Resuscitation in infants and children is an alarming thought, but do stress that when given promptly and properly it can save young lives. We never cease to be amazed at the apparent resilience of infants and young children. Children who seem to suffer the most appalling conditions or the severest of accidents have an amazing capability to come bounding back to a full, rich and normal life. To have played a part in saving the life of a young child must be one of the most rewarding human achievements.

PUTTING IT ALL TOGETHER

Anyone who has actually been involved in rendering emergency aid will be well aware that, in the heat of the moment, the urgent need is not so much for fragments of information as for an overall plan, a scheme of things into which the component sections can slot. In 'putting it all together' it is useful to offer your students a flow chart which they can learn and readily recall. Catchphrases and mnemonics (*aides memoires*) are also useful. The summary course of action recommended by the Resuscitation Council (outlined in a free colour poster from Vitalograph Ltd, see p. 150) is as follows:

Assess the scene
Assess the casualty
Is the casualty conscious? – Shake and Shout
Yes – reassure the casualty
    – check breathing and circulation
    – send for help
No

Airway
Open the airway by head tilt
Support the airway by chin lift
If airway obstruction is obvious – remove it.

Breathing
Look, listen and feel for breathing
Is the casualty breathing?
Yes – turn the casualty into the recovery position
    – check the airway, breathing and circulation
    – apply the rules for bleeding and shock if necessary
    – send for help
No – give four quick full breaths to fill the lungs. This may trigger breathing.

Are the breaths easy to get in?

No – this implies airway obstruction – deal with as
   appropriate. Re-check the breathing.

Yes – if the initial breaths are adequate but breathing
   does not re-start look for an underlying cause →

Circulation

Is there a pulse?

Yes – A non-breathing casualty who has a pulse should
   be given expired air resuscitation at the rate of
   about fifteen breaths per minute.

No – No breathing, no pulse means cardiac arrest.
   Commence cardiopulmonary resuscitation with
   two full breaths given between every fifteen
   compressions (eighty compressions per minute).
   (With assistance: five chest compressions to one
   breath.)

Check for a pulse after the first minute and every three
minutes thereafter.

If a spontaneous pulse does not return, prepare to continue CPR until skilled help arrives.

If a pulse returns, continue expired air resuscitation as
above.

If a pulse and breathing return, treat as for unconsciousness by placing in the recovery position.

This scheme is the basic outline of emergency aid and
resuscitation. The catch-phrases 'shake and shout';
'look, listen and feel'; 'CPR' act as reinforcers.

   The above may be considered as a *sequence* approach
and is the one favoured by the doctors and educationalists in the *Save A Life* organisation. An alternative
approach, valuable for breaking up the teaching class
and introduced originally by the Brighton Heart Guard
Scheme is the '*situation*' approach, ie what to do if . . .
Each situation is treated completely in itself before
moving on to the next one.

● The conscious casualty, eg someone having a heart attack or an asthma attack.

This covers getting help, warning signals, action plan.

● The unconscious casualty who is breathing.

This would include a road accident, poisoning, drunkenness, epileptic fit, etc.

Covers recovery position and shock.

● The unconscious casualty who is not breathing but has a pulse.

This includes drowning, gassing, head injury, etc.

● The unconscious casualty with no breathing and no pulse.

This covers cardiopulmonary resuscitation for a cardio-respiratory arrest.

This approach is sometimes useful but does suffer from the lack of cohesiveness – attention is drawn to the parts whilst obscuring the importance of the whole.

A B C or C A B ?

In Holland the sequence approach taught is different. It is known that people whose circulation stops from a heart attack remain well oxygenated up to the moment of cardiac arrest and, indeed, may continue breathing for a little while thereafter. For this reason the Dutch propose that chest compressions should precede attention to the airway and breathing. The initial chest compressions might provide a mechanical stimulus to restart the heart rather like the chest thump. In the well ordered environment of the hospital coronary care unit where it can be assumed that heart attack is the predominant cause of the arrest, then this approach may be effective. Anywhere else the cause of the arrest cannot be assumed and so we feel the time-honoured ABC approach is more logical. Certainly the ABC sequence is easy to remember and it is surely safer where laymen are concerned in that the dangers of applying external chest compressions when they are not appropriate are reduced.

One of the commonest findings of educational psychologists who examine resuscitation procedures is that people forget to feel for the pulse. Whatever the scheme of learning – ABC, CAB or Situation Instruction – *do remember to stress the importance of ensuring that the pulse is absent before commencing chest compressions.*

Some common questions

Students often ask the question 'at what stage in the resuscitation sequence can I go for help?' Their fear is that the casualty might be dead when they return. This fear of leaving the patient is countered by the feelings of panic that first aid helpers experience when they are stuck on their own doing something unfamiliar and slightly abhorrent with no one to support them. You cannot give hard and fast rules to your students because every case is different and, if they are stuck on their own, it really becomes a matter of judgement as to when is the safest time to leave the casualty. Certainly the full ABC sequence should be tried first. An unconscious casualty in the recovery position can be left unattended for a few minutes. Deciding whether to interrupt CPR on a cardiac arrest victim in order to seek help is very much a 'calculated risk'.

Similar anxieties are reflected in the question 'When should I stop resuscitation?' The answer is – do your best. If CPR is performed properly it can be given for a reasonably long time without fatigue. You should usually be able to continue until skilled help arrives. Otherwise go on until you are exhausted. If you have done all that you could as well as you could no one can criticise you for not doing more.

TRAINING MANIKINS

TYPES OF MANIKIN

Manikins are fundamental to the teaching and learning of practical skills in cardiopulmonary resuscitation. While practising mouth-to-mouth resuscitation on each other is not harmful (though hardly very agreeable), performing chest compressions on a normal subject whose heart is beating can be positively dangerous.

A variety of training devices with differing features exist but all have certain characteristics in common:

a) a means of 'opening the airway' by tilting back the head;

b) the facility to apply a tight seal to the mouth and/or nose for expired air resuscitation and to demonstrate adequate ventilation by causing the manikins' chest to rise with the inflation. With insufficient pressure applied or an air leak the chest should not rise;

c) the ability to allow demonstrably adequate chest compressions by producing a carotid pulse. The contour of the chest with the costal margin, xiphisternum and sternal body must be accurately simulated.

Some manikins have the ability to demonstrate the anatomy of resuscitation; some allow the stomach to inflate with incorrectly administered expired air resuscitation; some indicate wrong hand position or abnormal pressure applied to the chest; some simulate a means of dealing with a choking emergency. Some have been adapted for water rescue and emergency training for near-drowning. (Recording manikins are discussed on pp. 83–85.)

Manikins may be either an accurate anatomical facsimile of a patient ('life-like') or an obvious dummy; they may be full body or head/chest torso versions. To provide a change in 'feel' by using different types of manikins is quite important – organisers of classes could be encouraged to hold representative samples whilst probably settling for one sort for routine use. As an instructor you should try out and get to know as many different types as possible.

The degree of sophistication of manikins is reflected in their cost. Although the market is extremely competitive and devices are priced realistically, the choice depends upon the individual's needs and his pocket. The following notes give working descriptions of the major manufacturers' products used in the UK. For specific details you will need to read the manufacturers' operating manuals.

Resusci Anne (Laerdal Medical)

Resusci Anne is the best known training manikin; it was introduced in 1960 by Asmund Laerdal, a Norwegian toy and doll manufacturer. The manikin is extremely life-like and based on the body of a teenage girl dressed in a track suit. The face was modelled by sculptress Emma Mathiassen from the death mask of a young unknown girl pulled from the River Seine in Paris at the turn of the century. Many millions of people have practised CPR on Resusci Anne.

Expired air resuscitation on Resusci Anne may be performed through the mouth or through the nose. The mouth has teeth of a natural appearance and there is a connection between the mouth and nose. Air may pass through the manikin's airway when the head is bent forcefully backward or moderately backward combined with lifting of the jaw. Unless one of these methods is used the soft air tube will remain kinked. Inflated air passes through a hard air tube in the base of the neck to a corrugated tube connected to a non re-breathing valve. This directs air to a disposable lung located inside the manikin – as the lung is filled the chest wall rises. When inflation ceases the lung will empty and the chest fall down to its resting position. The air flows out of the lung back to the non re-breath-

79

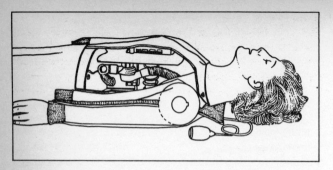

ing valve and is then directed out through a port in the manikin's right side.

When the sternum is depressed by external pressure the vertical movement is transferred to a piston located under the lower part of the sternum. When the pressure is released the chest will rise to its original position by the spring located around the cylinder and the compressing piston.

Anatomic Anne

Anatomic Anne is a torso manikin that shows all the relevant chest anatomy: a natural sternum, a cross section of the chest, lungs and heart with a simplified blood circulation system. Her head and upper airway are identical to those of Resusci Anne. Anatomic Anne is used to demonstrate and train people in both artificial ventilation and external chest compression.

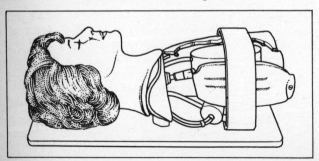

Resusci Baby
Resusci Baby is an infant resuscitation manikin with natural appearance, size and weight. It is used to teach and practice the special cardiopulmonary resuscitation techniques needed for infants.

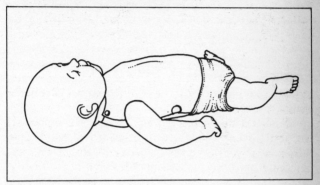

Resusci Junior
Resusci Junior is a new model from Laerdal designed to bridge the gap between Resusci Anne and Resusci Baby. Based on the body of a five-year-old boy, it has the special features of being able to float or drown. CPR can be performed in water or on dry land. It is becoming extremely popular for water safety and rescuer training.

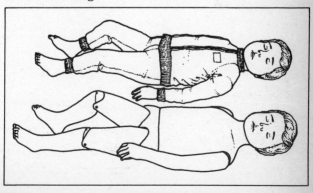

The Ambu Simulator

This is a torso dummy with a long neck, the good physiological features of which compensate for the lack of anatomical realism. The main feature of the Ambu manikin is a hygienic system by which means the expired air of the trainee inflates a disposable airbag in the model's head. This action forces the air already in the hermetically sealed head – but outside the airbag – down into the lungs. Each trainee has his 'own' face piece which is plugged into the disposable airbag in the head. The airbag and face piece are thus the only parts which come into contact with the expired air of the trainee. The head and neck section has a built-in valve and separate connections to the lungs and stomach. If the head tilt and chin lift is being performed incorrectly, expired air resuscitation will fail to inflate the lungs but cause the stomach to rise instead. A too high inflation pressure will also show as inflation of the stomach. Chest compression to a depth of $1\frac{1}{2}$–2 inches (4–5 cm) in the appropriate part of the chest will produce a carotid pulse in the neck. Pressure over the xiphoid results in a clicking sound simulating a fracture. A T-shirt illustrated with an anatomical drawing of the heart and lungs is available to fit over and protect the skin of the torso.

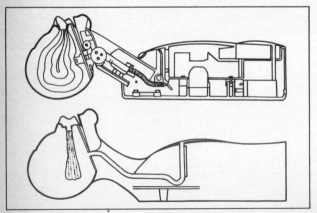

The Vitalograph Resuscitation Trainer
(C P Arthur)

This new manikin represents a middle-aged man of caucasian origin and is available in either torso or whole body versions. A simple single-user face piece (consisting of mouth/nose and throat) ensures that there is no risk of contamination. The 'lung' vents to the atmosphere through a one-way valve.

Expired air resuscitation can be performed by the mouth-to-mouth or mouth-to-nose method. The dummy has a 'rib cage' and chest compression will be permitted with correct head positioning. Both the lung volume and degree of head compression are adjustable to allow simulation of resuscitation on victims of various ages. All indicator circuits are pneumatic. The carotid pulse is generated by a squeeze bulb. One pupil is dilated; the other normal.

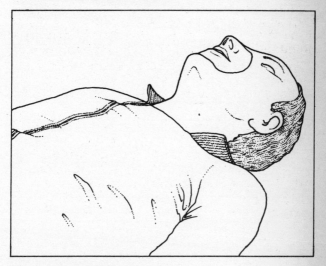

Recording manikins

Recording manikins have the ability to indicate in some manner the correctness and efficiency of cardiopulmonary resuscitation.

Laerdal manikins

These utilise an electronic light box which has the following signals:

GREEN for ventilation. When lung inflation volume reaches 800 ml (correct lung volume) the green light comes on.

YELLOW for compression. Depression of the *correct* part of the chest the *correct* distance (4 cm) activitates the yellow signal light. Overcompression (more than 5 cm) switches the light off.

RED for hand position. Sensors are located on the switch cover mounted on the underside of the chest cover. The red light will be activated if the chest is depressed with hands placed *outside* the correct area.

The Recording Resusci Anne has a built-in battery-operated paper chart recorder. This has three horizontal segments for registering inflation, compression and simulated pulse, and marking incorrect hand position. The recording paper is moved at an even speed and has vertical markings for time. The picture at the top shows a 'perfect' rhythm strip whereas that on the bottom shows a poor performance strip with several of

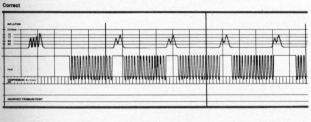

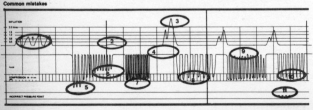

the common errors displayed. As instructors you should become familiar with the representation of such errors on recording strips. You will then be able to evaluate your students' efforts accurately, giving praise where possible and highlighting faults where necessary.

Ambu manikins
Each Ambu simulator has an outlet in the shoulder for plugging in gauges which indicate the volume of breathing effected (ventilation meter) and the depth and rate of compression achieved (blood pressure meter). Whereas the Laerdal system uses electronic signals, the Ambu gauges are pneumatic – that is they rely for their action on the pressure of air. Kinking or twisting in the connecting tubes will cause the gauges to give a false reading. The CPR Recorder is a mains-driven pneumatic chart recorder which can connect to the manikin with or without the other two gauges. The print-out chart provides an accurate record of the student's performance.

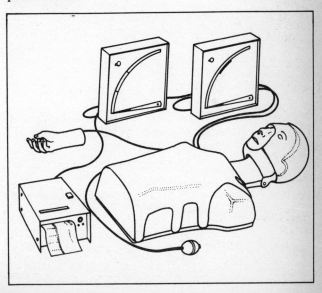

Care and maintenance of resuscitation manikins
Manikins are not toys – but they should be cared for with affection and respect. Ideally each instructor would have his own manikin which would then become his individual concern. More frequently, however, manikins are the pooled responsibility of a training scheme or society. Such an organisation probably has an equipment officer with the task of checking and maintaining the stock who will hold a number of essential spare parts and be responsible for ordering consumables, eg lung bags and chart recorder papers, etc. The officer probably also operates a booking system for the loan of manikins. However, the presence of an equipment officer does not absolve the individual instructor from any responsibility for manikin care. *Never* put a manikin away in its case dirty or incomplete. Always bring any faults immediately to the attention of the officer concerned. You will realise the importance of collective care the first time you pick up a manikin that someone else has left in an unsatisfactory state! Do read and *follow* the manufacturer's instructions. The resuscitation training equipment companies take great trouble over their after-sales service and follow up any complaints individually. Difficulties encountered are often simply a result of bad practice – the equipment itself is invariably sound.

HYGIENE IN TRAINING CLASSES
Learning resuscitation, as well as being enjoyable and satisfying, is inherently safe.

'To our knowledge the use of CPR training manikins has never been documented as being responsible for an outbreak or even an isolated case of bacterial, fungal or viral disease' (American Heart Association 1985).

Even so the general public do get squeamish and are apprehensive about performing mouth-to-mouth on models. There is no room for complacency. Hygiene in the use of manikins must be scrupulous.

1 Read the manufacturer's recommendations and provision for cleaning and disinfecting thoroughly.

2 Students and instructors should not work with a manikin if:

● they have skin lesions on the hands, mouth or face,
● they are hepatitis antibody carriers,
● they have AIDS,
● they have sore throats or colds,
● they have reason to believe that they have been exposed to, or are in the active stage of any infection.

3 Students should be assigned in small groups (ideally in pairs) to only one manikin – this lessens the possible contamination of several manikins by one individual and therefore limits possible exposure of other class members.

4 Ensure people follow basic rules of hygiene:

● thorough hand washing prior to contact with manikins or other students,
● no eating during class so as to avoid contamination of manikins with food particles,
● no smoking during class,
● remove lipstick before contact with manikins.

5 Manikins should be inspected regularly for signs of physical deterioration especially cracks or tears in plastic surfaces (for example, around the lips and nose) which make thorough cleaning difficult or impossible. The clothes and hair should be washed periodically.1?

6 If two-man CPR is to be practised the second student taking over ventilation on the manikin should simulate ventilation instead of actually blowing into the manikin.

7 Finger sweeps should be simulated or only performed on a specially prepared manikin.

8 At the end of each class the procedure listed by the manufacturer for thorough cleaning/disinfecting and drying outside and inside the manikin should be followed.

a) Take the manikin apart as directed in the manufacturer's instructions.

b) Thoroughly wash all external and internal surfaces

with warm soapy water and brushes. Thorough mechanical cleaning (scrubbing or wiping) is an extremely important first step in the de-contamination routine.
c) Rinse all surfaces with fresh water.
d) Wet all surfaces with an appropriate disinfecting solution. The choice of disinfecting solution has recently become the subject of much discussion. The Laerdal disinfecting fluid is perfectly adequate for the purpose, but expensive. It contains a mixture of alcohol and chlorhexidine (Hibitane). Hibitane on its own is not adequate and if the container is handled casually it could in time itself become a source of infection. The Center of Disease Control in the United States and the DHSS Communicable Diseases Surveillance Centre recommend the use of a sodium hypochlorite solution having at least 500 parts per million free available chlorine. In this country there is no statutory regulated strength of sodium hypochlorite (liquid household bleach). It is advisable to use 10 ml (two teaspoonsful) of bleach per pint of fresh cold water. In the form of Domestos, one of the strongest and most stable household bleaches available commercially, this provides 1800 parts per million free available chlorine. (The apparently excessive quantity of free chlorine allows for deterioration in strength during the period of its use, but at the same time is not strong enough to be objectionable in smell or residual taste.) If cheaper and weaker forms of commercial household bleach are used, the 10 ml bleach per pint of water still provides sufficient parts per million free available chlorine. The solution must be made fresh for each class and discarded after each use. The surfaces of the manikin must remain wet with the disinfecting solution for at least ten minutes. Laerdal provide a disinfection kit with their manikins and describe a method of cleaning and irrigating the dismantled manikin head after training sessions. Because bleach solutions, with repeated use, destroy the colour of the exterior of manikins, the manufacturers recommend that bleach solution be

used for the internal parts and disinfectant fluid reserved for the skin.

e) After a minimum of ten minutes, rinse with fresh water and immediately dry all external and internal surfaces. Rinsing with alcohol will aid drying of internal surfaces and this drying will prevent the survival and growth of bacterial or fungal pathogens.

9 Each time the instructor demonstrates a procedure and each time a different students uses the manikin, the face and inside of the mouth should be wiped vigorously with clean absorbent material, eg 4 in × 4 in gauze pad wetted with the alcohol/chlorhexidine solution. The surface should be allowed to remain wet before being wiped dry with a second piece of clean dry absorbent material. Alcohols alone are not ideal for this procedure as they may not be effective against bacteria or other pathogens in a short contact period. However, if you wet a piece of clean absorbent material with alcohol, instead of using a dry piece of material as mentioned above, and rub the area vigorously with this, the alcohol will act as a useful aid to mechanical cleaning and will help remove the odour of hypochlorite which some people find unpleasant.

Laerdal are introducing a new system to reduce the possible contamination of their manikins during use and to simplify their hygiene by the availability of disposable lower airways.

Face shields

Individual face guards, one to each student, may be used to ensure no cross-contamination takes place when performing mouth-to-mouth resuscitation. Each time a different student uses the manikin, the individual protective face shield should be changed. Ready-made protective plastic masks are available from Laerdal and new disposable face shields are being introduced.

Individual face pieces made of rubber or PVC are an integral part of the Ambu safety system described above. An illustration provided shows how to fit and

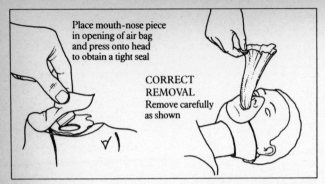

Place mouth-nose piece in opening of air bag and press onto head to obtain a tight seal

CORRECT REMOVAL Remove carefully as shown

remove the mouth/nosepiece and airbag. The rubber mask piece can be autoclaved or disinfected in boiling water. The PVC mask piece requires different treatment:

'On completion of the entire training session trainees should dispose of their used to a sealed bin or garbage bag and then de-contaminate their face/nose piece as follows:
1   Clean each face/nose piece by scrubbing for at least thirty seconds using a nailbrush, soap and running cold water.
2   Rinse the face/nose piece thoroughly with clean water.
3   Soak each face/nose piece in a disinfecting solution of 70% chlorhexidine for at least two minutes. Alternatively, soak in a 30% solution of alcoholic chlorhexidine for 1 hour.
4   Rinse thoroughly in water and allow each face/nose piece to dry thoroughly.
Decontaminated and dried face/nose pieces may be stored ready for next usage by replacing them in a clean container or plastic bag.'
(Recommendations of The Australian Resuscitation Council, December, 1985)

The detailed procedures given in this section may be felt by many instructors to be overcautious and unnecessary. We believe image to be all-important. If members of the public see their instructors taking care with their manikins and following sensible safety precautions as prevention against cross-infection, they will be suitably impressed and feel more secure. Recruitment to training classes should therefore increase.

TEACHING ADULTS

TEACHING ADULTS

There is no mystique about teaching adults – most of the 'rules' are commonsense. However, this is not to say that it is always easy to do, particularly for people who are only teachers in their spare time. Sometimes, the class can go disastrously wrong.

It was supposed to be about first aid in an emergency, but it turned into a harangue about road safety: very boring.
I didn't feel involved at all.

The instructor tried to teach us as if it was a military operation. He wasted endless minutes fussing over details, so several people, including me, never got to practise on the manikin at all.

I felt more confused at the end than at the beginning. It just seemed like a jumble of numbers, plus elaborate warnings about what could go wrong. I felt that as a result of the class I was probably less likely to offer help if someone collapsed than I had been before!

It's only fair to say that such comments are the exceptions, but they do show the importance of thinking hard about how to deliver an experience which adult students will enjoy and find useful.

Most of us can remember school days where teachers certainly taught away vigorously, but we sat with politely attentive faces masking minds that were far away. The teacher was 'teaching' but no-one was learning. The best definition of the difference between the two processes was given by the American educationists Postman and Weingartner. They commented dryly that to say you had taught someone something but they hadn't learnt it was about as logical as a salesman claiming that he had sold something to a customer who hadn't bought it. If the class does leave students feeling bored and frustrated, the fundamental reason is usually that the tutor has failed to understand this critical distinction between 'teaching' and 'learning'. The answer to someone who asks 'how can I improve my *teaching*?' is to suggest they change the question to 'how can I help my students *learn* more?'.

When a teaching session goes awry, there are three possible explanations. The first is that the tutor did not do the meticulous preparation that might have helped make it a success. The second is that the tutor has misunderstood the degree of authority his role gives him. He dominates and even bullies the class, usually by talking too much. The third possibility is that the tutor's nervousness and fear lead to apologetic and unassertive behaviour which students interpret as lack of interest and enthusiasm. All these problems can be overcome. How to prevent them arising in the first place is the subject of the following sections.

WHAT DO ADULT STUDENTS NEED?

Real learning always involves change: a change in skills, a change in attitudes, a change in knowledge. The only reliable way that such change can be brought about is for students to be thoroughly involved in their own progress. The skilful teachers are the ones who know how to make this happen because they are so well attuned to what their students need.

1 Relevance

Few people enrol to learn CPR out of a vague wish to improve their general knowledge. Students come either because they have already been involved in a situation where CPR was necessary or because they think that one day they might be. Students will expect your presentation to be vivid, practical and intensely relevant to their everyday lives. They have not come to learn detailed anatomy and physiology, nor to have 'improving' lectures on the prevention of heart disease, how to give up smoking, the history of the ambulance service, or

driving safely, though there might be a place for all
these topics in a different kind of course. The more you
can emphasise the everyday relevance of CPR skills, the
more closely they will listen.

2 Reassurance

Adults can make prickly, anxious learners. Many people
associate being a learner with the lowly status they
remember from school.

Becoming a learner again, even for a single evening,
may produce feelings of discomfort and uncertainty.
Will I look stupid? What if I don't do it correctly?
Most first aid instructors are rightly sensitive to this
possibility:

I always give people a chat at the beginning about it not
mattering if they don't succeed with the manikin straight
away. If that does happen, I offer to give them separate
practice at the end so that they don't feel silly in front of
each other.

It is important for people to preserve their dignity. If I spot
someone with badly fitting dentures, I know they won't get
a good result on the doll straight off. I have a tactful word
with them privately about ways round the problem.

3 Activity and involvement

Most CPR teaching and learning has to be crammed into
little pockets of time in busy lives: perhaps a lunchtime
session at the workplace, or more commonly, a few
hours in the evening at the end of a long day. Many
students, however keen and interested they are, will be
tired. They are likely to find concentration difficult,
especially if there are long stretches of monotony and
passive listening in the class. The more active learning
there is, for instance, practising the recovery position in
pairs, practising mouth-to-mouth breathing on the
manikin, or a general discussion – the more this problem will recede. The more variety of pace and teaching
media you can build in, the better the response will be.

Active learning is important for another reason. The only significant way that adults and children differ as learners is that short-term memory facility declines in adults. In everyday life this shows itself in irritating little lapses: for instance, looking up an STD code and then finding that you have forgotten the telephone number that goes with it. What has happened here is that looking up the code has 'interfered' with the 'storage' of the number in your short-term memory.

Translated to a class environment, this means that any 'teaching' involving more than a few minutes of verbally given instruction is likely to leave many students confused. This will be particularly true of the full CPR cycle where information about breathing rates, numbers of compressions a minute and numbers of cycles can come quick and fast, often to bewildering effect.

The solution is straightforward: adults learn best by *doing*. Being 'told' that the rate of compressions should be fifteen per minute will probably sail straight over the heads of many students. A student who herself counts to fifteen on the manikin is much more likely to learn the sequence successfully. This advice is often summed up in what is sometimes claimed to be an old Chinese proverb:

'I hear and I forget
I see and I remember
I do and I understand'

4   Practice, Feedback, Reinforcement
Research into learning has shown again and again that people learn most effectively when they have maximum opportunity to practise and reinforce whatever skill they are acquiring. This can often be a problem in CPR classes, especially if the numbers are large. If you have time, ask people who are uncertain to stay behind later. Encourage them to read the Campaign pamphlet as soon as they get home and to re-read it frequently.

Where CPR is concerned research has also shown how quickly the learning 'decays'. Many people have already forgotten a good deal of what they learnt after about six months. Remind students that 'refresher' courses are always a good idea: at least once every three years is probably the desirable minimum.

Students always need lavish feedback on their performance. Knowing whether or not you have done something successfully is an essential part of learning. Some manikins are capable of providing instant feedback (see pp. 83–85), ranging from red and green lights to a detailed printout. This is an excellent aid to student learning, but it should not prevent you adding more feedback of your own, ranging from a simple 'very good' or 'no, not quite . . . try again this way' to more detailed comment on a student's efforts.

People learn most quickly when they get a 'right' answer to a problem. The feeling of achievement is one of the best possible spurs to wanting to continue learning. It is commonly said that we learn by our mistakes. In reality, people thrive on success. The skill for tutors is to give people tasks which are just within their competence so that the possibility of making errors is minimal, while the task itself is just complex enough to retain the student's interest. This is particularly important with adults where mistaken first efforts have a way of lodging in people's minds. The lesson of this in teaching CPR is to teach a little at a time in a way the student is sure to get right. For instance, it is probably best to teach everyone how to open the airway and let them practise it as a discrete sequence before going on to the recovery position or mouth-to-mouth breathing and so on. Put the complete sequence together, of course, but only aim to do it as the final element.

5 Experience welcome!

In the sixties and early seventies, many towns and cities started 'community colleges' which often encouraged adults and teenagers to share the same tuition. To their eternal shame, some of the teachers involved, who were encountering adult learners for the first time, could be overheard complaining that the adults were a nuisance. Why? They would insist on questioning things and offering their own experience. . .

Adults have lived longer than children and therefore have more opinions and experience at your disposal as a teacher. Some of this may be a distraction, but much may be highly relevant to the group. Many people enrol for CPR training because they have been involved in a medical emergency; many groups will include people with some kind of medical training. Solicit their comment, use their experience, invite participation. The more involved people feel, the more they are likely to learn.

6 Pattern and Structure

Most things are easier to learn if we can see how they form a pattern. The 'ABC' structure of CPR is already a great help here. But on a broader level, always start by telling students exactly what your objectives are and how you will set about achieving them. Tell them that there will be practice sessions and a discussion session (if you plan one). If you have the time and resources give people a hand-out which outlines the programme for the evening. Either way emphasise from the start that you will teach CPR through the ABC mnemonic which will help them both learn and retain the sequence.

BEING A TUTOR

Most CPR classes meet only once and for a few hours. Nonetheless a high degree of skill will be demanded of you as their tutor. Your students will expect to leave the class confident that they would know what to do in a life-threatening emergency. Before this desirable conclusion is reached you will need to have displayed the social skills of a gifted host, the group-management skills of a professional psychologist, the communication skill and organizational talent as well as the good humour and authority of the perfect chairman. No wonder that some educationalists have claimed, with justification, that being a teacher is one of the most demanding and complex roles there is, exceeded in complexity only by the role of being a parent.

The irony of good teaching is that the better it is, the more unobtrusive it seems to become: the elated students tend to leave the class convinced that they have done it all by themselves.

Preparation
The room
A wise and experienced teacher of adults once gave it as his opinion that you could forget your fancy theories about teaching and learning: the most important thing was to get your room arranged properly, then you were pretty certain to have a successful class.

Perhaps this is an exaggeration. But it does contain a useful element of truth. Putting it the other way round, if you do not prepare the room suitably it will make your job much, much harder. Here are some examples from real life of the things that can go wrong:

An enormous unheated church hall with too many chairs all set out in straight rows; a dirty splintered floor. About twelve students present, but two left before the end of the class, complaining of the cold. No practice mats provided. To the tutor's dismay, several of the women refused to practise the recovery position, saying they were wearing 'best' clothes. All those who did laddered their tights.

A small room containing about fifty chairs left higgeldy piggeldy by the last occupants. Twenty students present. Much time wasted by chaotic and unsuccessful efforts halfway through the class to clear enough space for the practical part of the class.

Pleasant, clean, well-lit warm room. Chairs set out in five rigidly straight rows to accommodate sixty students. Discussion session at the end of the class a complete failure: only two people spoke, in spite of constant prodding from the tutor.

The size and shape of the room, the type of chairs and the way they are arranged are all hidden but powerful influences on the success or failure of a class. Of course, it is often the case that a tutor can have little choice but to make do with unsatisfactory accommodation. Even here, however, it is often possible to make significant improvements.

You can reduce the apparent size of an over-large room by setting out the chairs at one end of it. This is better than filling the space in the middle, which will emphasise the yawning gaps all around. In a small room, remove all the redundant chairs if you can.

A room with a dirty floor in poor condition is unsuitable for first-aid teaching and will justifiably be a cause of resentment to students. If you cannot provide mats or blankets, you should make every effort to find an alternative room.

Heating and ventilation can often present problems. Both over-heated and cold rooms will produce inattentive students. Be prepared to make adjustments if you can.

Seating arrangements
You will want the class to be successful as a social group, however fleeting its members' contact with one another. To help this happen, you must 'fine-tune' the seating pattern.

In everyday life, seating arrangements usually reflect status and personal feelings. A boss who wishes to draw attention to his own power will talk to a subordinate from behind a desk. A group which meets as a committee will usually leave plenty of space on either side of the chairman, thus emphasising his leadership role. A clergyman's special status with his congregation is underlined by the fact that he not only addresses people who sit in straight rows facing him, but also that he frequently does so from the elevated position of a pulpit: he literally is 'on high'. On the other hand, most of us have experience of the reverse pattern – sitting physically close to people usually produces feelings of comradeship, especially where plenty of eye-contact is possible. Think, for instance, of having to share a small table in a restaurant with complete strangers. In this situation, most of us feel a compulsion to exchange at least some friendly words.

You can use these basic rules of human behaviour to good effect in a class.

● Seat people in a circle whenever possible. This way they can see and hear each other better. It is also far less easy for shy people to hide. Another virtue of this seating arrangement is that you will have a much clearer view yourself of how individuals are feeling at any one time. If you want to demonstrate, it will be easier for people to observe.

● Circles are not a good idea for groups larger than twenty-five: the circle becomes straggly and the physical distances increase too much. Some kind of sitting-in-rows arrangement is probably inevitable with large groups. However, curving the rows will still be better than leaving them straight; two semi-circles of chairs will probably make people feel much more involved.

● Remove any redundant chairs. There will always be people whose instinct is to lurk in a corner. Ideally you want everybody to participate, so lurking must be discouraged. The simplest way to do this is to remove the potential hiding places.

● Arrangements sometimes go wrong at the last minute and you may inherit a room with too many chairs set out in an unsuitable way. Be ruthless about asking students to sit where *you* want them to. Most people react meekly when courtesously asked to bring their chairs forward, or to fill front seats.

● Push the chairs as close together as possible. This literally reduces the physical distance between people, but it also reduces psychological distance. People who are almost huddled together normally feel more friendly towards one another; the group begins to work as a *group* not just as a collection of individuals.

AUDIOVISUAL AIDS

Many lay people may only have hazy ideas of how their bodies work. Learning CPR may therefore present them with a number of difficulties. Of course you are not required to teach full-scale anatomy and physiology. On the other hand most people will absorb your information better if they know a little, for instance, about how the respiratory system works, or what the role of the tongue is in unconsciousness. It is often said that one picture is worth a thousand words, and teaching CPR offers a good example of the truth of the maxim.

Visual aids offer a change of pace and something different to look at. They have the further advantage that they show you have cared enough about your teaching to prepare carefully.

As a rough and ready rule, try to offer people a visual aid – a slide, a chart, a working model or a TV clip – about once every three or four minutes.

There is no doubt that appropriate visual aids, imaginatively used, greatly enhance the impact of any teaching. Equally, there is no doubt that poorly designed visual aids ineptly used can destroy everything you set out to achieve. We have probably all sat through exquisitely embarrassing occasions where the lecturer has had to shout over a noisy, badly focussed slide projector, where the promised 'video' is a snowy mess, or where a sad heap of new electrical equipment sits unused because no-one discovered in time that the room had old-fashioned round-pin sockets.

Proper preparation will dispose of most of the problems. First, think about why you want a visual aid at all; each one must earn its place on grounds of merit. The questions you need to ask are:

Is it a better way of explaining a process than words alone?

Is its graphic standard high enough?

Will it help produce a change of pace?

Will it help people remember the teaching point you want to make?

You should only go ahead if you can answer 'yes' to all these questions.

Next, you should consider the particular advantages of each type of visual aid.

Chalk boards are simple, informal, flexible and familiar. However, they do not produce exciting visual images, and they have the further disadvantage that to write on them during the class, you must turn your back, thus losing contact with the group.

Overhead projectors are a better way of doing the same job. The image is brighter and sharper, transparencies can be prepared in advance using special Letraset, felt tip pens or photographic processes. You can write on the plastic film during a class without turning your back. However, hastily hand-scrawled words or drawings can often look amateurish. Normally, it is better to prepare transparencies in advance.

Flip charts These large sheets of paper are really a paper version of the blackboard. The large white sheets lend themselves well to bright thick felt-tip pens. Again, material can be prepared in advance or you can write on them during the class.

Slide projectors A strong sequence of professionally made slides can be a powerful visual aid, often better and certainly much cheaper than home-made video of uncertain quality. For instance, one tutor produced an excellent set of ten slides taken at a road accident to prompt discussion on treatment of priorities. Another opens his session with an amusing sequence giving the history of methods of artificial resuscitation. However, it is rarely worth bothering with a slide projector unless your material is as punchy and competently produced as this.

Tape may be an excellent way of introducing local colour and relevance to the seassion. If you know of people who have been rescuers or successfully rescued, why not get them to tell their stories on tape? Many people who don't like the idea of providing publicity material for local newspapers, are quite happy to be anonymous voices for a class. Your local radio station might be prepared to help you produce and edit such a tape.

Video There are many CPR training videos on the market. Video material has many advantages. It can show demonstrations in close-up – often surprisingly hard to achieve in a class situation. It can have a power-fully arousing effect emotionally. It is a good tongue-loosener; everyone is used to giving their opinions about television programmes, and a video presentation will often succeed in prompting discussion where other methods fail.

However, it has many potential disadvantages too. Poorly made video material with unconvincing acting and leaden presentation may be rejected by a group used to higher standards of broadcast television. As a teaching medium it can never rival face-to-face tuition because its relentless pace will always be wrong for part of the group.

Don't look to video to do your basic job for you. You have the advantage of being able to spot what your class is finding difficult or easy to understand. Use video material for its capacity to arouse interest: per-haps by showing a short, scene-setting drama at the beginning of the class. You could use another extract again at the end: possibly the whole cycle of CPR as a reinforcement of what your group has just learnt.

Never take a video on trust: always preview, always select the extract you want.

Film is an older version of video. The disadvantages are that it must be projected by someone who is trained in using the equipment. Projectors can be noisy unless they are in a separate projection box; the film itself is fragile and easily scratched. On the other hand, film is probably better for large groups because it will provide better sound and picture quality.

Presentation

Most students are used to high standards of graphic presentation from their familiarity with poster-design and graphic sequences on television. It is worth taking some trouble if you are producing home-made visual aids. The main rules are:

● Keep it simple. Don't overcrowd each 'frame'.
● Use solid blocks of sharply contrasting colour whenever possible.
● Keep captions to a minimum, write them horizontally.
● Allow people time to absorb the meaning of each aid as you show it: pause a moment if possible.
● Dispose of each visual aid as soon as you have finished with it. For instance, students will find it distracting to be looking at a diagram of the respiratory system when the tutor has got onto the causes of a heart attack.

If you feel uncertain about your own ability to prepare visual material, there are many sources of potential help. All local education authorities employ audio-visual aids specialists, sometimes in teachers' centres, sometimes in schools and colleges. You may be able to make an informal arrangement whereby slides or OHP transparencies can be prepared for you. Similarly, if you are in contact with a local teaching hospital, you may be able to persuade their audiovisual aids unit to help you produce the material you want. Sources of commercially prepared material are listed on p. 147.

Housekeeping

Having planned and prepared the material itself, audio-visual aids demand their own housekeeping chores. Always double-check the booking if you are borrowing equipment. Who is to be responsible for bringing the equipment to the class? When will it arrive? Who will operate it? Are there spare bulbs available for projectors? Do the plugs and sockets match? Remember that a video may need re-tuning and leads may need reconnecting: if you are using video, make sure you familiarise yourself with this aspect of how they work. Are the leads to the equipment long enough? Do you need black-out? Is the equipment in good working order? It is mysterious how often a journey on a trolley down a short corridor produces non-functioning machinery: make sure you have allowed time to check everything on site before the group arrives. Finally, who will return equipment and lock it away at the end of the session?

CREATING THE ATMOSPHERE

Most of your group will be unknown to each other. Perhaps one or two will have come with a friend; if you are operating in a workplace then there may be groups of colleagues who arrive together. Basically, however, you must assume that you are working with a group who are strangers to each other. They are going to be required to touch each other in unfamiliar and possibly embarassing ways. The more you can create a relaxed, friendly, but purposeful atmosphere, the more quickly such difficulties will dissolve. Some ways of achieving this:

● Arrive at least twenty minutes early. This gives you time to double check audiovisual aids, prepare the manikin and to set out the room as you want it.

● Greet each person on arrival and make them feel welcome. If you have time, ask them what, in particular, has brought them to the class and whether they have learnt any first aid before. Possessing such information can be a useful way of drawing people in to the discussion later.

● Large name labels are useful, if funds permit. They will enable you to address people by name and will encourage group members to learn each other's names. Anything which makes people feel individually valued and recognised is useful. First names are more friendly than formal titles. Make sure you are wearing a name label yourself.

● Start and finish promptly. Nothing is more irritating to people who have arrived on time than to be kept hanging about for the people who are late. Inevitably, then, the class finishes later than scheduled, which may mean students miss buses or have to pay their baby-sitters overtime. Tell the class at the start what time you intend to finish and stick to it. Offer to stay later and give extra, informal tuition if you have time and the room is still available.

● Introduce yourself and say a few sentences about your own background. Students will expect you to have authority in your subject, but it never does any harm to fill in a few details. If you are working with several other instructors, introduce them all with a few words about each of them.

● You are in charge, so it is up to you to keep to a brisk pace, and to create a cheerful, workmanlike atmosphere. It is up to you to control the loquacious and encourage the silent. Don't be afraid of laughter: shaking a manikin and addressing it as a human being has an absurd side which most people relish. Laughter is a good way of reducing tension, so encourage it as long as it does not threaten your control of the group.

● Coffee and refreshments are another useful way of breaking the ice, especially at the beginning of the class. Of course this is not always possible in borrowed premises and with a tight timetable. But even instant coffee and powdered milk in paper cups can work wonders as a way of creating a friendly atmosphere. To organise coffee you will need a helper: your own attention must always go to the students.

PUTTING IT ACROSS

Giving a talk

We hope we have already shown that teaching CPR effectively is going to involve your class in a great deal of practical learning. Nonetheless, there is probably going to be a part of the class time when all eyes are on you because you may be giving a five-minute opening talk, a ten-minute explanation somewhere in the middle of the session, or a five-minute 'round up' at the end.

Few of us are gifted orators or natural raconteurs; most of us have been bored or embarrassed by people who know their subject but don't seem able to put it across well. Yet surprisingly enough, the rules of good spoken communication are simple. Applying them can make all the difference between a limp, inadequate talk and one that is clear, interesting and inspiring.

1 *Preparation*

Careful preparation underlies all good teaching. Make notes of all your main points, then reduce them to headings on a postcard which you can carry in your hand if you like. Don't be tempted to write yourself a script: you will end up reading it, which looks and sounds inappropriate for an informal occasion and emphasises any lack of confidence you may feel.

Most good tutors will confess to nerves before a class just as almost all actors feel some stage fright before a performance. Some tutors will say that it is almost worth carefully cultivating nervousness as it gives an edge to what they say. There is probably a lot of truth in this. A tutor's preparation should include a reminder that adult students are free agents. Coming to a class nearly always involves giving up various attractive alternative ways of spending their time. Just a little nervousness will help you put some zip into your talk. If you are too relaxed you could also be too dull.

2 Make the framework clear

First you tell them what you're going to tell them; then you tell them; then you tell them what you've told them.

This is a good rule for any teaching, but it applies especially to giving talks and lectures. Your talk should have a beginning, a middle and an end, and this framework must also be perceptible to your listeners.

Try to stick to five or six main points as this is usually the maximum people can take in. Tell people what the points are in advance and list them again as you come to them.

3 Speak enthusiastically

Many ill-prepared lecturers get away with murder because they speak in such an enthusiastic and lively way. The opposite can also be true: a tutor who has spent many hours toiling conscientiously on preparation can throw away his advantage by delivering his talk in an apologetic, sad mumble. Look lively, smile, keep your head up, sound keen on your subject. Effective teachers always convey enthusiasm: everything in their manner suggests an urgent desire to share their knowledge with their class.

4 Avoid jargon

CPR is part of medicine, therefore it is potentially full of technical words. Try to avoid all medical jargon except the few words you feel people must understand. Explain what technical words mean every time you use them.

The best communication is usually the simplest. Most lay people find long words and medical terminology off-putting. A student who is privately puzzling over whether 'ventilation' is the same as 'breathing' will probably have missed the next part of your presentation while he works out the answer.

5 *Keep it brief*

It is hard for adults to concentrate effectively for more than about twelve minutes of being 'talked at'. If you are tempted to go on for longer, ask yourself if the extra time is really justified. Much unsuccessful lecturing and talking is based on what we might call 'The Hole in the Head Theory of Education'. This is the one where the teacher assumes that students have a hole in the head through which 'knowledge' can be poured. Unfortunately, learning is not so simple. Talking uninterruptedly and at length only usually results in listeners' minds wandering far away from the subject of the class.

Try not to complicate your talk with too many rambling accounts of medical controversies or 'ifs' and 'buts'. Certainly give lively examples of dramatic rescues throughout your talk because they are a good way of capturing people's interest, but don't allow yourself to be sidetracked from the main points.

6 *Watch your mannerisms*

Many of us have no idea what our own mannerisms are. The more they take over speech and gesture, the more wildly irritating they can be to an audience. After all, your hearers are obliged to look at you: if you reduce your group to counting your 'ums' and 'ers' and the number of times you scratch your nose, you can be sure that they are not giving full attention to what you are saying. Try to keep mannerisms under control. The most common are: pacing nervously up and down, excessive throat-clearing, looking at the ceiling, jingling keys or coins, crossing arms, head-scratching. Most of these can be cured by standing at a table and holding it lightly with both hands.

7 *Eye contact*

Nervousness and inexperience lead many tutors to make the mistake of looking anywhere but at the students: at the floor, at some invisible object at the back of the room, at just one half of the group, or even worse, at just one individual. Keep sweeping the group with your gaze: that way everyone can feel that you are interested in them and you really want to communicate with them personally. Never make the mistake of turning your back on the group as this breaks eye-contact. If you use chalk boards or flipcharts, have them prepared in advance.

8 *Keep 'reading' the group*
Scanning the group has another virtue: it means that you are constantly observing your audience. An interested group returns your gaze, sits still, nods agreement and looks generally lively. But are they shuffling their feet or fidgeting with handbags? Are their faces blank and eyes glazed? Has anyone closed their eyes? Has whispering broken out at the back? If so, you have lost their interest and you must take drastic measures to re-engage it: stop and ask for comments perhaps, or better still, stop altogether and get on to the practical part of the class.

Demonstration
Demonstration is an invaluable teaching technique for CPR tutors. Nevertheless, it is important to remember that it is a *teaching* and not a learning tool. Just because you have demonstrated CPR, this does not guarantee that your students have learnt it. Indeed, demonstration has many of the same disadvantages as lecturing in that it too tends to be a one-way process. It must be consolidated immediately through practice if it is to be successful.

Good demonstrators usually keep to these rules:

● Simplicity. Stick to the main points. Don't clutter your demonstration with long accounts of difficult rescues, or 'ifs' and 'buts'.
● Brevity. Teach one short sequence at a time, then let people practise.

● Sightlines. Make sure everyone can see; encourage people to move if they can't. Normally it is better for people to have an over-shoulder view by standing behind you. That way they don't have to keep mentally reversing right and left hands.

● Keep looking at the group: don't make the mistake of addressing all your advice to the manikin or to the floor.

● Repetition, reinforcement. Aim to build up the correct sequence by constantly repeating the same information in the same order. Get the students to do the same when they are practising by repeating a verbal sequence.

Role-play

Role-play is a useful technique, which could perhaps be more widely employed than it is in teaching CPR. It involves students working in pairs or small groups and acting out a given situation. Some possible scenarios:

One student assumes the role of a casualty with heart attack symptoms. Her partner gives reassurance and support along the recommended lines.

Students practise calling an ambulance. One is given a piece of paper with details of the casualty (heart attack, road accident and so on). The other plays the person in the Ambulance Control Office (give this student a list of 'prompts').

Students practise dealing with a choking incident (without practising the Heimlich manoeuvre).

Role-play is a useful way of keeping all the students involved in active learning for as much of the time as possible. For instance, it can help solve the problems created by having a large group and only one manikin.

It is also a good way of learning how to deal with the taxing situations of real life. It enables students to practise in a 'sheltered' environment where it is possible to make mistakes without feeling silly. Nevertheless, it is not the answer to every teaching difficulty and does need to be set-up carefully if it is to be of maximum value in the class.

Making role-play work

● Tell students why you are using the technique and what you hope to achieve with it.

● Prepare carefully. It often helps to hand each student of the pair a separate briefing sheet with a few lines about the situation they are to role-play. For example:

You are Brian, a fifty-five year old man with no previous heart problems. During the last week you have felt tired and unwell and have been meaning to go to your GP. You are now at work – you have an office job – and in the last fifteen minutes you have been feeling acute pain in your chest which is now spreading to your left arm and jaw. You ask your colleague for help.

You are Sandra, a colleague at Brian's office. It's a small firm with no nursing staff, though there is a qualified first aider on the premises. You have noticed that Brian has not been looking well for a few days. The time is just after lunch. He tells you that he feels ill. What do you do?

● Reassure students that no great acting ability is required – it is a rehearsal of procedures, not an audition for a part in a play. Nonetheless, you may find some students too shy and self-conscious to take part. Accept their refusals gracefully.

De-briefing

Role-play should always be discussed, either by the pair involved or, preferably, by a large group. How did the role-play go? If you had been the casualty, would you have been reassured? Was the advice or information given clearly? Has anyone been in a real-life situation like the one portrayed? If, so, was it different? Is 'textbook' advice always feasible in reality?

A useful variant on role-play is a discussion based on a brief case study. As with role-play, this technique probably works best with a small group of between four and six people. The idea again is to present students with some of the 'what if . . . ?' dilemmas of real life. These are probably best written down and distributed individually so that students have the details in front of them. Here is an example:

You are driving north on the M1 in your black Metro with a friend. It's 11 o'clock at night, winter, and raining heavily. You suddenly come upon the scene of an accident. An Escort saloon and some kind of tanker have collided. The tanker is in the slow lane, the Escort is slewed across the middle lane. What do you do?

Discussion

Most CPR classes benefit from a period of discussion, usually at the end of the session. Valuable though this can be, it is as well to be clear in your own mind about why you are introducing a discussion and what you expect to achieve from it.

Don't for instance, confuse genuine discussion with a question-and-answer session designed to test what students have retained from the session. If this is your aim you would be better off with a light-hearted quiz or a printed 'test yourself' questionnaire which students can take away with them and check against the *Save A Life* Campaign pamphlet or the *First Aid Manual*.

Discussion is ideally suited to two particular tasks where CPR is concerned. First, it gives people the chance to clear up any lingering factual confusions. Secondly, and probably much more importantly, it is the time when they can explore the feelings involved in being a rescuer. Here discussion is an ideal teaching method as it works best in situations where there are no 'right' or 'wrong' answers and people can learn from each other.

Some first aid tutors concentrate exclusively on CPR techniques in their classes. They feel that in the short time available it is more important to drum home the 'facts' than it is to enter the grey and perilous area of emotions.

In favour of this kind of discussion, however, is a good deal of anecdotal evidence from students that it contributes considerably to the enjoyment and meaning they get from the class. Many people enrol for CPR training because they have felt helpless and ignorant at the scene of an emergency. Others may have tried to give help in an incident where a casualty has died. The powerful emotions of confusion and guilt generated by such events probably need to be dealt with publicly if students are to feel they can cope 'better' next time and apply the knowledge they have acquired in a class.

Furthermore, it is only fair to warn students that being a rescuer in real life is a tense and possibly messy experience, nothing like practising CPR on a sterile manikin in the pleasant environment of a first-aid class. It is probably better for such information to come from other students than from the tutor as it will have more authenticity and the students who offer their experience will feel gratified that they have contributed valuable material to the group. The class itself will become a more interesting and enriching event because of the variety and quality of contributions made by its members.

It is difficult to run an effective discussion with a group that is too large. The ideal size is somewhere between eight and fifteen. A smaller group may not produce enough variety of experience. With larger groups a rule of inverse participation operates: the bigger the group, the smaller the number of people who speak, perhaps because it takes an unusually self-confident person to cope with the large number of people.

The seating pattern (see p. 100) is also important.

It is difficult to promote good discussion if people cannot see and hear each other. A 'discussion' where people sit in straight rows will always tend to turn into a question-and-answer session with the tutor capping every comment from a student. In a true discussion the comments will cross the group with only occasional discreet comment from the tutor.

Achieving useful discussion

It was once the fashion to sneer at the use of discussion in education as 'a pooling of ignorance'. This, perhaps, is a good description of discussion inappropriately employed by an unskilled tutor. In the right hands and to the right ends it is a superb technique and probably the only truly effective way of changing attitudes. So how good discussion be achieved?

● *Be clear about objectives* Have in your head the two or three main points you want the group to explore. These might be questions like

How would you feel about giving CPR to a complete stranger?
Is it appropriate to visit a resuscitated casualty later?
How would you feel if the person you help dies?

Your objective should be to guide students to uncover some of the difficulties and dilemmas of real life, not to impose your own view. If they seek guidance from you, then of course you should answer honestly, but your main purpose should be to solicit contributions from the group. Tell the group that this is your intention and explain why.

● *Allow for pauses and silence:* Silence need not be threatening. A thoughtful pause often makes it easier for a shy person to get in to a discussion and makes it clear that measured comment is more welcome than quick smart answers. Be especially alert to the danger of following every comment from a student with one of your own. If you say anything, let it be of the 'would anyone else like to add anything?' variety.

● *Clarify:* Be ready, however, to clarify confused and stumbling contributions by re-phrasing them, or relating them to earlier parts of the discussion.

● *Be alert to the possibility of emotional distress in some group members:* An apparently neutral question or comment might mask a painful personal experience. For instance, in one group, a young student asked whether GPs should be called first rather than an ambulance to heart attack patients. The carefully phrased and tactful answer showed that the tutor had drawn her own conclusions from the bleak face of the questioner. Sure enough, further discussion revealed that this student's father had recently died an hour after his GP had been called and then had left in the middle of the night.

● *Control:* Be ready to control the discussion by steering it discreetly in new directions where necessary.

● *Don't hesitate to interrupt:* An over-confident and noisy student may sabotage all your attempts to persuade everyone to participate. Avoid his eye and, if that doesn't work, don't hesitate to be politely ruthless, if necessary by actually talking across him, or saying 'Thanks, but I'd like to hear from someone else now'.

● *Draw out:* Silent members should be encouraged to speak. Some ways of doing this are:

Ask general questions but look in the direction of someone who has not spoken.
Say 'Is there anyone who hasn't contributed yet who'd like to comment?'

Beware of appearing to pick on people unless you know that they are likely to have views on a topic. Singling them out may simply make them feel more uncomfortable and even less likely to contribute again.

● *Sum up:* This is not, of course, the opportunity for you to hold forth about your own views. Rather it should be a skilful summary of the main views expressed. A summary is important; it reinforces the idea that discussion is valuable and it emphasises that there is no 'correct' opinion on such difficult topics.

SAVE A LIFE
(HEC BOOKLET TEXT)

We have reprinted here the text (but not the illustrations) of the student booklet produced by the Health Education Council for the *Save A Life* Campaign.

This booklet is distributed free to everyone who attends a class.

BASICS

YOU HAVE THREE MINUTES

When a casualty has stopped breathing, the brain can only survive for about three minutes without oxygen. So don't waste time: every second counts. Of course it is frightening to be a bystander in an emergency, but you can learn the simple ABC routine which will help you remember what to do:

APPROACH

Approach carefully and make sure you are not in any danger yourself.

ASSESS

Assess the situation. It is vital to assess the casualty quickly and accurately.

IS THE CASUALTY CONSCIOUS?

Shake the casualty gently and shout 'Are you all right?' An unconscious person cannot respond. If the casualty is unconscious you must start the **A B C** routine without delay.

A AIRWAY

IS THE AIRWAY OPEN

A blocked airway prevents breathing, causes unconsciousness and may lead to death. If the airway is blocked, you must open it.

B BREATHING

IS THE CASUALTY BREATHING?

If breathing has stopped you must try to restart it by giving mouth-to-mouth breathing.

C CIRCULATION

DOES THE CASUALTY HAVE A PULSE? IS THE CASUALTY BLEEDING?

The blood may have stopped circulating around the body because the heart has stopped beating.

If this has happened the casualty will not have a pulse. You must try to restart the circulation by giving chest compressions.

If the casualty is bleeding you must control it as soon as possible.

APPROACH

There are, unfortunately, many cases where a bystander trying to be helpful has also become an accident victim. There is little point in heroism if you involve yourself and others in danger unnecessarily. The rules are:

Electricity

Never touch a casualty who is still in contact with the electricity supply. Turn off the current and remove the plug before attempting emergency aid.

Gas or poisonous fumes
Keep clear if you cannot cut off the source and
ventilate the area properly.

Fire
Many accidents involve fire risks from spilled
petrol or escaping gases. Turn off the ignition
in a crashed car. Don't allow anyone to smoke.

Road accidents
If you are driving, park your car safely behind
the crashed car. Ask another bystander to direct
the traffic round the accident and well clear of
the casualty and yourself. Turn on your hazard
lights and use a hazard triangle if you have one.

Assess

IS THE CASUALTY CONSCIOUS?

It is vital to assess the casualty quickly and
accurately. Shake the casualty gently and shout
'Are you all right?' An unconscious person
cannot respond. If the casualty is unconscious
you must start the ABC routine without delay.

CALLING FOR HELP

When you are alone and first on the scene you
should always treat the casualty before doing
anything else: delay can be fatal. Then call the
emergency services as soon as you can,
especially in these cases:

- unconsciousness
- difficulty in breathing
- suspected heart attack
- severe bleeding
- serious burns

Emergency calls are free.

Dial 999. The Emergency Operator will answer, saying 'Emergency, which service do you want?' Ask for an ambulance. The Emergency Operator will ask for your phone number and will put you through to the ambulance service.

Be prepared to pass on the following information:

● Your telephone number, in case you are cut off.

● Exactly where the incident has occurred. Include the name of the road, house number and any landmarks that might help the ambulance find its way.

● What has happened: how many people, the kinds of injuries they seem to have.

Ambulance Control has direct contact with other emergency services and will alert the police and fire services if necessary.

Don't replace the receiver until the ambulance control officer has done so: he or she may need to ask you more questions.

A AIRWAY

Hundreds of otherwise healthy people die unnecessarily in accidents, not from their injuries as such, but from a blocked airway. If you have established that the casualty is unconscious you must open the airway. It may be blocked because in an unconscious person lying on his back, the tongue becomes floppy and blocks the airway.

Opening the airway

1   Place one hand under the casualty's neck to

support it. Put your other hand on his forehead. Gently tilt his head backwards.

2 Now push his chin upwards. Lifting the jaw like this brings his tongue forward, and opens his airway.

3 In many cases, opening the airway will be enough to allow breathing to restart, even though the casualty may still be unconscious. If breathing does restart, turn him into the recovery position and stay with him until help arrives.

THE RECOVERY POSITION

This is a safe, stable and comfortable position for all unconscious casualties who are breathing and whose hearts are beating. Placing the casualty in the recovery position makes sure that the airway stays open. The tongue cannot fall back into the throat, and vomit can drain away freely.

1 With the casualty lying on her back, kneel beside her level with her chest. Turn her head towards you and tilt it back slightly to open the airway.

2 Bend the arm furthest away from you and lay it across her chest.

3 Place the arm nearest you by the casualty's side then slide her hand palm upwards underneath her buttock.

4 Cross her further ankle over her nearer ankle.

5 Support the casualty's head with one hand. Use the other to grasp the clothes at the hip furthest away from you.

6 Gently roll the casualty towards you until she is resting against your knees.

Readjust her head to make sure that her airway is open.

7   Bend the casualty's uppermost arm and then her uppermost leg. This stops the casualty rolling on to her face.

If necessary ease out her other arm and leave it lying parallel to her back. This stops her rolling back.

Neck or spinal injuries

Take particular care when using the recovery position if you suspect neck or spinal injury. Always suspect spinal injury in:

- road traffic accidents
- falls from ladders or down stairs
- horseriding accidents
- rugby scrum mishaps
- dives into shallow water

In such cases, don't over-tilt or twist the head. Keep the head and neck in one line and get at least three others to help you turn the casualty in a 'log roll' on to their side.

B   BREATHING

Look, Listen, Feel

Is the casualty breathing?

LOOK at the chest: does it rise and fall? Put your ear over the casualty's mouth and LISTEN. If she is breathing you should be able to hear her breath. Can you FEEL her breath on your cheek? A casualty who is not breathing may have a bluish tinge inside her lips (this is noticeable whatever skin colour the casualty has).

Clearing the airway

1   If she is not breathing her airway may be blocked by a foreign body. Turn her head to one side, keeping her chin well up.

2   Hook your index finger and use it to sweep quickly inside her mouth and pull out any foreign matter, for instance loose teeth, weeds, vomit.

3   Leave well-fitting false teeth in place.

Mouth-to-mouth breathing (ventilation)

An unconscious person who has stopped breathing will die within a few minutes unless you can get air into the lungs. Mouth-to-mouth breathing ('the kiss of life') is an effective way of doing it. This 'rescue breathing' is effective because the air you breathe out yourself contains enough oxygen to keep a casualty alive.

Don't waste time: every second counts

1   Open the airway. Clear it if necessary. Keep the casualty's head back and the chin held upwards.

2   Pinch her nostrils and keep them closed tightly. Maintain this 'seal' or the air you blow in will escape through her nose.

3   Open your own mouth wide and take a deep breath.

4   Seal your lips tightly round the casualty's mouth.

5   Blow into the casualty's mouth. The blowing should be gentle but firm and the chest should rise.

6   Remove your mouth and allow her chest to fall.

7   If the chest does not rise and fall, you must assume that the airway is not properly open. Try tilting the casualty's head back more and lifting the chin.

8   Check that you have pinched the nostrils firmly enough and that your lips are tightly

sealed round the casualty's mouth. If the chest is still not rising and falling, the airway may be blocked by a foreign body.

9   Repeat this cycle giving four rapid, full breaths. Watch the chest to make sure it rises with each breath. These four quick breaths may be enough to restart breathing.

10   If breathing does not start, check the pulse to make sure that her heart is beating. If the heart is beating but breathing still has not returned, continue the mouth-to-mouth breathing at the rate of about 15 breaths a minute.

11   When the casualty starts breathing normally again, you should turn her into the recovery position. This is because a resuscitated casualty will often vomit and the recovery position will prevent her choking on the vomit.

CHILDREN

If you are a parent you will want to know how to deal with the kind of serious emergency that might threaten your child. Fortunately, heart attacks are extremely rare in children. However, children are still at risk from accidents in the home, on roads or in water, any of which may lead to airway and breathing problems.

The basic techniques of emergency aid are the same as for adults, but they must be done slightly faster and with much lighter pressure.

Young children and babies

1   Seal the child's *mouth and nose* with your mouth and blow gently into her lungs until the chest rises.

2   Breathe at the rate of 20 breaths per minute (every three seconds).

Note: Only practise mouth-to-mouth breathing on specially-designed 'manikins' under a tutor's supervision in a first aid class.

C CIRCULATION

Chest compression
The casualty's airway has been opened and he has been given mouth-to-mouth breathing. If he is still not breathing his heart may have stopped and you need to get it beating again. You can make it pump blood by rhythmically pressing on his chest: this is called external chest compression ('heart massage'). Without this help, blood carrying oxygen cannot reach the brain and there will be permanent brain damage after only a few minutes.

Don't waste time: every second counts

1   Check the pulse in the casualty's neck by sliding your fingers between the Adam's apple and the thick, firm muscle running up the side of the neck. No pulse means the heart has stopped beating (the casualty has had a 'cardiac arrest').
2   Make sure the casualty is lying on his back preferably on a firm surface. Kneel beside him. Feel for the breastbone: it runs down the centre of the chest from the collar bones to the last pair of ribs.
3   Put the heel of one hand on the lower half of the breastbone. This is where the heart is.
4   Cover this hand with the heel of your other hand and lock your fingers together.
5   Lean forward, keeping your elbows absolutely straight. The combination of straight

arms and locked hands will allow you to press down in the most effective way.

6   Press down firmly on the breastbone. You should aim to push the chest down $1\frac{1}{2}$ to 2 inches (4–5 cm). Then at once release the pressure.

7. Keep pressing rhythmically on the chest. Count 15 compressions by saying out loud 'One-and, two-and, three-and . . .' until you reach 15.

8   Move back to the casualty's head. Re-open the airway and give two breaths through the mouth, sealing the nose as before.

9   Continue this cycle. You should aim for about 80 compressions a minute, giving them in cycles of 15 compressions followed by two mouth-to-mouth breaths.

10 Check the pulse after the first minute (four cycles), then every three minutes.

11 When the pulse returns, stop chest compression. Continue mouth-to-mouth breathing until breathing starts again.

When the casualty has a pulse and is breathing normally, turn him into the recovery position. Keep checking breathing and pulse until medical help arrives.

Giving chest compression is tiring. But it is vital to continue the whole cycle of mouth-to-mouth breathing and chest compression (cardiopulmonary resuscitation, CPR for short) until skilled help arrives. If you are tired, get another bystander to take over for a while.

Note: only practise chest compression under a tutor's supervision on a manikin in a first aid class.

STOPPING BLEEDING

Heavy loss of blood can lead to shock and to death. Serious bleeding can often be simply controlled.

● Lay the casualty down. This gets more blood back to the heart.
● Press over the wound with thumb and fingers.
● Raise the injured limb above heart level. It may take several minutes for bleeding to stop.
● Cover the wound with a dressing. Ideally this should be sterile, but improvise with any clean, non-fluffy material if necessary. If blood seeps through, add more dressings on top without removing the original one.

Shock
Shock can follow severe bleeding. The symptoms are:

● Feelings of faintness and anxiety
● Pale, clammy skin
● Shallow breathing
● Weak pulse
● Vomiting

Shock is dangerous and can lead to unconsciousness and death.

● Reassure and comfort the casualty.
● Lay him down.
● Raise his legs: this helps the blood supply to the brain.
● Keep him warm (but not with a hot water bottle or by rubbing, which will draw blood away from the vital organs).

● Turn him on to his side if he starts to vomit.

Important : Don't under any circumstances give him anything to drink. It might make him vomit. Also, he may need an anaesthetic later.

HEART ATTACKS

A 'heart attack' means that the flow of blood to the muscles of the heart has been blocked.
If you suspect a heart attack, your main aims should be :
● to call an ambulance as soon as possible
● to do everything you can to look after the casualty until skilled medical help arrives.

The signals
● an uncomfortable feeling of pressure ; gripping fullness or pain in the centre of the chest which may spread to arms, neck, throat, jaw and back
● breathlessness
● a feeling of weakness or giddiness
● paleness, heavy sweating, and sometimes blue lips and finger tips.
A heart attack is often preceded by several days of feeling overwhelmingly tired and generally unwell. There may have been chest pain dismissed as 'indigestion'. It is unusual for very severe chest pain to come on suddenly. Typically it develops over several minutes.

Don't waste time : every second counts

1 Dial 999 and call an ambulance immediately. Say you suspect a heart attack.
2 Offer reassurance and comfort.
3 Ask if he would like tight clothing loosened.
4 Help him get comfortable. Half-sitting,

half-lying with shoulders supported and knees bent is often a good position, but let him choose.

5   Keep checking pulse and breathing.

6   If he loses consciousness, keep checking his pulse and breathing. If there is no pulse you must start mouth-to-mouth breathing and chest compressions and continue until medical help arrives.

CHOKING

This alarming and potentially fatal emergency happens when food, vomit or an object such as a broken tooth, a sweet or bead goes down 'the wrong way'.

Don't waste time: every second counts

1   Reassure the casualty and encourage her to try to cough. The efforts to cough may be enough to dislodge the obstruction.

2   Sweep a hooked finger around the mouth. This is sometimes enough to remove the object.

3   If that fails, tell her to bend over: gravity will help. Slap her sharply between the shoulder blades about four times. In almost all cases, this will be enough and the object will shoot out of the throat.

4   As a last resort, *and only if everything else has failed*, you can try 'abdominal thrusts'. Stand behind the casualty and put one arm around her stomach. Clench your fist.

5   Grasp your fist with your other hand.

6   Pull sharply inwards and upwards. You are pushing the upper abdomen against the lungs. This will drive air upwards and force out the blockage. Repeat up to four times. The obstruction may then shoot out of the mouth.

If, in spite of help, the obstruction remains and the casualty becomes unconscious, open the airway and try mouth-to-mouth breathing.

Small children
Sit down and lay the child over your knee, head down. Slap him sharply between the shoulder blades four times. Use a little less force than you would use for an adult.

Babies
Lie the baby along your arm, head down. Slap him smartly but lightly between the shoulder blades.

ROAD ACCIDENTS

Thousands of people die every year in road accidents. Many of these lives might have been saved if someone at the scene had known what to do.

When you approach a major road accident you should ask yourself:

● Is the accident scene safe? Am I putting myself at risk from other traffic?
● Are there hazard warning signs on lorries and vans? These indicate dangerous chemicals so be very careful.
● How many casualties are there? Some may be trapped, some may be wandering, dazed, a distance away.
● Who is most seriously injured? Someone making no noise at all may be much more seriously hurt than a casualty who is shouting for help or moaning.

● Who can go for help? Someone should call the emergency services immediately.
● Try to give a simple job to people who are panicking: this will help calm them down.

1 Protect the area from other traffic. Park your own car well away from the accident, behind it if possible. Turn on your hazard lights and set up a hazard triangle if you have one. At night use something light coloured to make yourself visible. If you are wearing a dark jacket, take it off.

2 Ask another bystander to direct traffic away from the accident.

3 Turn off the ignition in the crashed cars: this reduces the risk of fire.

4 Diesel lorries and buses often have an emergency fuel supply switch outside the vehicle: switch it off.

5 Check that handbrakes are on.

6 Look inside vehicles for small children who might have rolled on to the floor or been thrown out of sight. Ask a conscious casualty how many people were in the car.

7 Do not move casualties unless there is danger of fire. The ambulance services are trained in the special techniques needed to move and transport injured people.

8 A trapped casualty must be watched carefully. If he becomes unconscious his tongue may fall to the back of his throat and block his airway.

9 In this case, open his airway by supporting and extending the neck until the ambulance arrives.

10 Deal with victims in this order of priority:

- unconscious, not breathing
- bleeding severely
- unconscious but breathing
- conscious but shocked.

DROWNING

Most deaths from drowning occur at unsupervised rivers and canals. Swimming pools and beaches are safer. However, even here, you could be involved in an emergency where your help could be vital.

Important: Remember the golden rule of giving help: don't endanger yourself or others unnecessarily.

- Send for professional help as soon as possible.
- Think about your own safety. If possible, stand in a safe place on dry land from where you can give clear, calming instructions.
- Most swimming accidents occur within a few yards of the bank where it would be possible for a rescuer to reach out or throw something (eg a lifebuoy rope, or piece of wood) to the victim.
- Don't attempt a swimming rescue unless you are a competent swimmer trained in life-saving. The sudden shock of cold water, the danger from rocks or of struggling with the panicking victim could turn you into a casualty yourself.

Treating an apparently-drowned casualty

- Don't waste time trying to empty the lungs of water; this is unnecessary.
- Sweep the casualty's mouth clear of weeds or other obstructions and open his airway.

● If breathing has stopped, start mouth-to-mouth breathing immediately. If there is no pulse, start chest compression.
● When breathing and pulse return put the casualty in the recovery position and keep him warm.
● Call an ambulance. All casualties rescued from drowning must be sent to hospital, as there is a danger of lung congestion which may develop several hours later.

BEING A RESCUER

Being present at an emergency and giving first aid is not a neutral experience. It is much more likely to be an event which lingers on in the mind vividly and perhaps uncomfortably. Did I do the right thing? Could I have done more? This is particularly the case if the person you rescue appears ungrateful or if the casualty dies in spite of your help.

If you have been involved in an incident of this sort, you should bear in mind that you can only do your best given your knowledge and the circumstances at the time. For instance, you are unlikely to know all the facts of the case. If someone dies, it may well be that even the most prompt, skilled medical assistance could not have saved their life. The important thing is that you tried to do something, even if it was only calling the ambulance.

Learning first aid in a class, in a pleasant environment, on a clean manikin, is very different from the tense and probably messy circumstances of real life. It is not surprising, then, that some people who have given help reproach themselves afterwards with not having done it 'properly'. Again it is better to think positively. You did something. It may well be that what you did was the only possible course of action given the situation at the time.

Many people enrol for a first aid class after they have felt helpless at an emergency. This is a positive and direct way to deal with the experience. You at least have the reassurance that you will be better equipped to cope next time.

Important

First aid skills do need constant practice if they are to remain clearly in your head. Try to go on a 'refresher' course at least once every three years. Keep this booklet in a place where you can re-read it frequently and refer to it easily.

THE SAVE A LIFE CAMPAIGN

The *Save A Life* Campaign is one of the most important initiatives ever to be made in the area of community health in the United Kingdom. The campaign has two objectives:

1 To raise the general level of public awareness as to how to sustain life in an emergency;

2 To persuade many thousands of people to undergo practical training in emergency aid.

In its design and execution the campaign satisfies the four criteria identified by Dr Peter Safar in his book *Cardiopulmonary Cerebral Resuscitation* as being essential for a successful national resuscitation campaign:

- medical consensus
- guidelines
- public awareness
- implementation

Medical consensus

The campaign is being conducted under the solid aegis of the Royal Society of Medicine with Sir John Walton as Patron. Active support and encouragement has been pledged from:

Department of Health and Social Security
Department of Health and Social Security Welsh Office
Scottish Home and Health Department
Health Education Council
The British Medical Association
The British Heart Foundation
The British Association for Immediate Care
The Resuscitation Council of the United Kingdom
The Royal College of General Practitioners

The Royal College of Physicians of London
The Royal College of Physicians of Edinburgh
The Royal College of Surgeons of England
The Royal College of Physicians and Surgeons of Glasgow
The Royal Life-Saving Society
The Casualty Surgeons Association

The rationale for the campaign 'that a knowledge in the community of the major principles of emergency aid would produce a substantial reduction in the number of sudden deaths from respiratory obstruction and cardiac arrest' emphasised in the Introduction to this book has been accepted by the medical profession represented through these bodies.

Guidelines

The views expressed in this book reflect the guidelines of the *Save A Life* Campaign committee which includes senior advisers from the three major Voluntary Aid Societies of the United Kingdom and the Resuscitation Council. The guidelines are believed to be scientifically accurate and educationally sound. The curriculum for a single session course in resuscitation and emergency aid is described on pp. 141–143. The techniques will be taught according to the third impression of the 4th edition of the *First Aid Manual* (St John, Red Cross and St Andrew's, 1982).

Public awareness

The campaign centres around six BBC Television programmes being broadcast at peak times starting in October 1986. The programme contents are as follows:

Programme 1 – Opening the Airway (and Road Traffic Accident)
Programme 2 – The Recovery Position
Programme 3 – Mouth to Mouth Breathing (and Drowning)
Programme 4 – CPR

Programme 5 – Recognising the Signs of a Heart Attack

Programme 6 – Choking

The TV programmes are being accompanied by the distribution of associated campaign literature designed and produced by the Health Education Council.

A quarter of a million booklets for the *That's the Limit* campaign were distributed through surgeries, hospitals, community centres and Health Education departments. There are similar intentions for *Save a Life.* Free posters provided by the Laerdal Company exhorting people to come forward for classes will be distributed for display in every town and village in the United Kingdom.

The Health Education Council's Report *Health Education in the Mass Media* suggests that it is appropriate to implement a mass media campaign when the desired behaviour is a single action – writing a letter, attending a clinic or using a telephone. The *Save A Life* Campaign fits well into known successful models of Health Education using the media. The same viewing audiences as for previous campaigns are confidently expected. The campaign also aims to persuade viewers to write for free leaflets. There will be further encouragement to responders to attend classes since considerable publicity from national and local press and radio is expected.

Implementation

The co-ordination of the campaign is vested in the Campaign Director based at the Royal Society of Medicine. All queries, requests for leaflets, and classes by the television will be handled by Broadcasting Support Services. This is a support agency highly experienced in dealing with mass requests of this kind. They will send each enquirer a leaflet containing the address of a local centre and details of classes. These organisers will set up classes, co-ordinate instructors and will respond to any direct enquiries. The model adapted is that of the Adult Literacy Campaign. About 120 local centres spread across the nation are the requirements. These will usually be provided by the Local Education Authority (LEA) who are well used to organising and managing adult education classes.

Each local centre will hold lists of training facilities, potential trainers and location of manikins. Lists of local classes plus their contacts, telephone numbers and addresses will be sent from a national base to the local centres. It is then intended that the local referral organisers can make further contact with the public and set up training sessions in response to local requirements. The training at local level is being provided by:

Red Cross
St John Ambulance
St Andrews
Royal Life Saving Society
Swimming Teachers' Association
Ambulance Service
Police
Armed Services
The 15–20 already existing local schemes.

The local centres will hold quantities of 24-page booklets (upon which this Instructors' Guide is based) which will be given to each attender of the course. A charge of about £2 per trainee is recommended to go towards training costs and to provide an honorarium to assist instructors with out-of-pocket expenses.

The campaign gives an unparalleled opportunity, never before available in this country, to study and evaluate a national campaign involving links between Health and Education. Not only will the sampling techniques enable an assessment to be made of the numbers of people in this country with first aid knowledge, but it will also be able to quantify the effects of that knowledge in terms of action undertaken by members of the public and by the number of lives saved.

The *Save A Life* Campaign management is massive. The organisation problems have been colossal. Yet at the time of publishing this book the signs are of a highly successful and worthwhile outcome. At the end of the day and the end of the line it will be each individual instructor who will influence the quality and extent of that success.

SAVE A LIFE
CORE CURRICULUM

The following is the formal advice being given to local organisers for the curriculum and content of a single-session training class within the *Save A Life* Campaign.

Curriculum for a single session course in Resuscitation and Emergency aid

A 'class' will normally last $2-2\frac{1}{2}$ hours, the exact timing depending upon local arrangements, local needs and the availability of instructors. Execution of CPR training in a single session demands the use of adult resuscitation training manikins – a ratio of six students per instructor/manikin (maximum ten) is optimal. Variations in the course organisation (eg attention to road accidents, heart disease prevention, alteration of student/instructor ratios) are permitted provided that the minimum content is covered as follows:

1 Introduction to the course

The brain's need for oxygen is discussed with brain damage occurring after a few minutes oxygen lack. The need is demonstrated for a clear **A**irway, adequate **B**reathing and intact **C**irculation. 'Resuscitation' is defined as the reversal of deficiencies in these areas. A wide variety of emergencies may present with the same fundamental problems and similar principles used which are common to them all.

2 Priorities

The first priority is safety – to self and victim. The rescuer must exclude or eliminate danger, eg road accidents, electricity, fire or gas etc.). Then a careful approach to the casualty should establish unconsciousness by shaking gently and speaking loudly. Avoid further damage to other injuries, eg neck and back, by unnecessary movement.

Someone is sent to get help – knowledge of the 999 system is important.

3 The airway

The causes of airway obstruction are discussed – in particular the role of the tongue in unconsciousness and airway obstruction due to foreign body (food, blood or vomit). The airway is opened by tilting the head back and supporting the jaw/chin. The choking emergency is dealt with by finger sweeps and back blows.

The recovery position is described and practised.

4 The breathing

The student is taught to look, listen and feel for breathing: the causes of absent breathing including (particularly) drowning and gassing are described. The techniques of expired air resuscitation by the mouth-to-mouth/mouth-to-nose methods are practised. The student is taught to give four initial breaths to inflate the lungs: if still no response to check the circulation. A casualty who is not breathing but who still has a good pulse rate is treated by mouth-to-mouth breathing at 15 breaths per minute.

5 The circulation

The components of the circulation – the Pump (Heart) and Pipes (Blood Vessels) are described. The nature, causes and recognition of a heart attack are described. Bleeding from arteries and veins is described. The student is taught to feel for the carotid pulse and the importance of recognising an absent pulse is stressed. When the heart has stopped (cardiac arrest) there will be no pulse and no breathing. Both breathing and circulation are supported by mouth-to-mouth breathing and external chest compressions (cardiopulmonary resuscitation or CPR). The student must demonstrate proficiency at single handed CPR (fifteen compressions at eighty per minute followed by two breaths). The pulse is checked after one and each third minute. The chest thump is not taught.

At the discretion of the instructors two-man rescue may be demonstrated (5:1 at sixty per minute) but time usually precludes student practice at two-man resuscitation.

The rules for bleeding are discussed – laying the casualty down, raising the affected limb and applying direct pressure over the wound by pad or grasping. The shocked patient must be insulated from a cold environment and not given anything by mouth – the position for protection from cold should be demonstrated with a blanket *under* the casualty.

6 Children
The essential difference in resuscitation between children and adults is the respiratory nature of the emergency. Some causes of asphyxia in children and their management are discussed (choking, suffocation, inhalation etc.). Expired air resuscitation by the mouth-to-mouth and nose method may be demonstrated (especially if a baby/child manikin is available). Chest compressions are not taught in children.

7 Resumé
The above may be described by way of example in a practical setting. The way in which the different aspects of first-aid are coordinated are explained in order to overcome the student's anxieties and inhibitions.

It is stressed that the course is the bare minimum required to learn how to 'save a life', that refresher training is desirable in the future and that complete first aid courses are available through voluntary aid societies.

Techniques according to: 3rd impression of 4th edition of *First Aid Manual* (St John, Red Cross and St Andrew's).

SOME NOTES ON AIDS

Many people are worried that by performing mouth-to-mouth resuscitation they will put themselves at risk of becoming infected by a severe life-threatening disease – in particular AIDS. Such worries are reinforced by an awareness of the fact that the virus which causes AIDS may be found in the saliva of infected subjects. To reassure people (and yourself), some background knowledge about AIDS will probably be useful.

What is AIDS?

AIDS is the end result of a virus infection. This virus, known as HTLV-III (Human T-cell Lymphotrophic Virus type III) likes to live in special white blood cells called T-lymphocytes. These are the cells which usually prompt the body's defence mechanism, the immune system, into action causing it to switch on and off appropriately when infection attacks.

As viruses cannot survive without cells, the HTLV-III virus (it is not called the AIDS virus) needs to come into contact with body fluids containing a high white cell count before it causes infection. It is a frail virus and repeated contacts with high concentrations of virus are needed before infection occurs. White blood cells are most heavily concentrated in blood and semen and are present in tears or saliva in low concentrations. This is why no cases of AIDS have been passed on through tears or saliva.

Transmission of the virus occurs most commonly (1) between homosexuals, (2) with intravenous drug abusers and (3) in cases of transfusion of contaminated blood products. The illustration shows the time scale in which the virus, having invaded the body may, rarely, go on to produce the condition AIDS. Less than one per cent of those originally infected with HTLV-III will

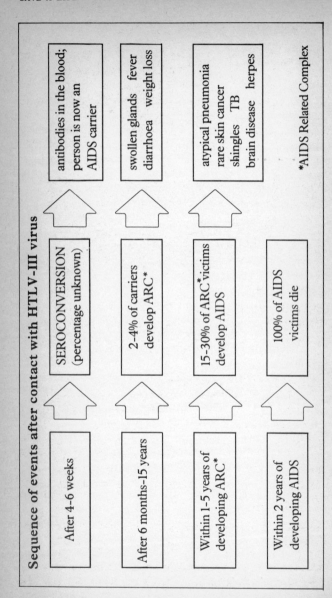

Sequence of events after contact with HTLV-III virus

After 4-6 weeks → SEROCONVERSION (percentage unknown) → antibodies in the blood; person is now an AIDS carrier

After 6 months-15 years → 2-4% of carriers develop ARC* → swollen glands   fever   diarrhoea   weight loss

Within 1-5 years of developing ARC* → 15-30% of ARC* victims develop AIDS → atypical pneumonia   rare skin cancer   shingles   TB   brain disease   herpes

Within 2 years of developing AIDS → 100% of AIDS victims die

*AIDS Related Complex

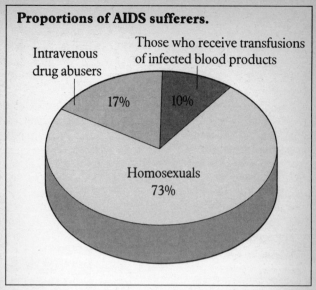

Proportions of AIDS sufferers.

Those who receive transfusions of infected blood products

Intravenous drug abusers

17%   10%

Homosexuals
73%

actually develop AIDS. The commonest conditions which finally kill an AIDS patient are an unusual type of pneumonia, a rare skin cancer, shingles, tuberculosis and thrush.

The size of the problem
The disease has been studied most closely in the USA. It probably did not exist before 1970. At the current time there may be one million people infected with the virus in the United States and it is expected that 1–2% of them will develop the disease over the next year. In the UK there are 20 000 people with the HTLV-III virus, 287 recorded cases of AIDS with 144 deaths reported by February 1986.

Is there a risk of contracting AIDS from CPR?
There is no known link between CPR and AIDS.

In the USA where the AIDS epidemic is higher than in the UK, your chance of contracting AIDS through giving CPR

145

is less than one in a million. Compare this with the one in 5000 chance of dying in a car accident, one in 10 000 chance of being murdered. Giving CPR to a casual contact will not increase this risk. Remember, eight out of ten people who give CPR do so in the home to people they know, not to a high risk stranger.

The unknown victims of arrested breathing (near drowned children, middle-aged heart attack casualties, etc.) that people might have to deal with are unlikely to be in those groups of patients who are carriers of AIDS. Health care workers who might have to apply resuscitation on a very regular basis or who, in the course of their professional duties, might come into contact with high risk groups, would be expected to take special precautions against disease transmission by using bag and mask or other interposition devices. Even then, the only recorded case of a health professional contracting AIDS was that of a nurse who actively injected herself with blood from an AIDS victim. A case of exposure to the AIDS virus in CPR has been reported recently when two nurses in North Carolina gave mouth-to-mouth resuscitation to a haemophiliac known to have AIDS. Regular and repeated blood tests were carried out on these nurses for nine months and *all the tests were totally negative* for any sign of virus transmission.

RESUSCITATION AND FIRST AID TRAINING MATERIAL

Audiovisual sources

The following organisations distribute audiovisual material (slides, 16 mm films and video cassettes in various formats). They all have first aid material in their catalogues. Many offer facilities for previewing. Telephone first to ask for a catalogue and for booking information.

BBC Enterprises Limited
Education and Training Sales
Woodlands
80 Wood Lane
London
W12 0TT
Tel: 01-576 0519/0237

Produce a pack containing two video cassettes (VHS) bearing the complete *Save A Life* television series, a copy of this book, a pamphlet about the campaign and a copy of the HEC student booklet. Also produce video cassettes of the *Mind How You Go* road accident prevention series, the last programme of which describes emergency procedures at a traffic accident.

British Heart Foundation
102 Gloucester Place
London
W1H 4DH
Tel: 01-935 0185

Camera Talks Ltd
31 North Row
London
W1
Tel: 01-560 0762

Eothen Films Ltd
EMI Film Studios
Shenley Road
Boreham Wood
Herts
Tel: 01-953 1600

Graves Medical Audiovisual Library
Holly House
220 New London Road
Chelmsford
Essex
CM2 9BJ
Tel: 0245 83351

Guild Sound and Vision
6 Royce Road
Peterborough
PE1 5YB
Tel: 0733 315315

Holiday Brothers (A/V) Ltd
172 Finley Lane
Heald Green
Cheadle
Cheshire
SK8 3PU
Tel: 061-437 0538/9 or 061-436 4780

Edward Patterson Associates Ltd
Treetops
Cannongate Road
Hythe
Kent
C21 2PT
Tel: 0303 64195

Rank Aldis Educational Films and Video
PO Box 70
Great West Road
Brentford, Middlesex
Tel: 01-560 0762

School Traffic Education Programme
2309/11 Coventry Road
Birmingham
B26 3TB
Tel: 021-742-4296
Produce a film and video called *Killing Time* (11 minutes) on how to proceed at a road traffic accident and first-aid priorities generally.

Stewart Film Distributors Ltd
107–115 Long Acre
London
WC2E 9NT
Tel: 01-240 5148
Have a new programme called *ABC of CPR* made with St John Ambulance for the Royal Navy. It is available at a special price to *Save A Life* instructors.

Videotel Marine International
44 Great Marlborough Street
London
W1V 1DB
Tel: 01-439 6301

Viewtech Audiovisual Ltd
161 Winchester Road
Brislington
Bristol
BS4 3NJ
Tel: 0272 773422

Computer Software

P. M. Burridge
Consultant Anaesthetist
Birch Hill Hospital
Rochdale
OL12 9QB
Rochdale Health Authority has software on teaching CPR available on cassette for the BBC Microcomputer. It is free of copyright and transferable to disc. Enquiries to the above address.

Manikin Manufacturers

Ambu International (UK) Ltd
Charlton Road
Midsomer Norton
Bath
BA3 4DR
Tel: 0761 416868
Produce the CPR Simulator with options of head section
model, pulse simulator, recording gauge, chart re-
corder, anatomical T-shirts.

Laerdal Medical Ltd
Laerdal House
Goodmead Road
Orpington
Kent
BR6 0HX
Tel: 0869 76634
Laerdal produce the 'Anne' range of manikins together
with an extensive range of first aid training aids. They
are UK agents for Pyramid Films (USA) which pro-
duces, amongst others, the film *CPR for Heartsavers*
with excellent graphics and sequences. Their 'Group
Trainer' comprises flipchart easel, instructor guide,
groundsheet and kneeling mat, students' notes etc.
together with video copy of the above film.

Vitalograph Ltd
Maids Moreton House
Buckingham
Bucks
MK18 1SW
Tel: 0280 813691
This film produces the new Resuscitation Trainer
'C. P. Arthur' with accessories. It distributes free of
charge the A3 Resuscitation Council wall poster and
has the British video *ABC of Resuscitation* available
for sale.

Off-Air Educational TV Recordings

It is legally permitted to make sound and videotape recordings of BBC and ITV educational programmes within certain copyright limitations.

Details about forthcoming school and further education series and information about the copyright limitations can be obtained from:

Villiers House
The Broadway
London
W5 2PA
Tel: 01-743 8000

Head of Educational Programme Services
Independent Broadcasting Authority
70 Brompton Road
London
SW3
Tel: 01-584 7011

Voluntary Aid Societies

The British Red Cross Society
9 Grosvenor Crescent
London
SW1X 7EJ
Tel: 01-235 5454
This society produces a programme *First Aid for Life* in four parts.

1 Emergency
2 As I live and breathe
3 Blood loss and shock
4 Bones can break

Available for hire or sale through Guild Sound and Vision (film or video) or on loan to member branches together with other approved training material, posters and wall charts available from Head Office.

St John Ambulance
1 Grosvenor Crescent
London
SW1X 7EF
Tel: 01-235 5231
St John have no audiovisual material of their own but make recommendations to member branches on the suitability of commercially available material (see below).

St Andrew Ambulance Association
St Andrews House
Milton Street
Glasgow
G4 0HR
Tel: 041-332 4031

Swimming Teachers Association
Aquatic Rescue Division
Anchor House
Birch Street
Walsall
West Midlands
WS2 8HZ
Tel: 0922 645097

Royal Life Saving Society UK
Mountbatten House
Studley
Warwickshire
B80 7NN
Tel: 052-785 3943
This society produces a set of illustrations as colour transparencies, OHP vu-foils or flip charts based on the current edition of the 'Resuscitation and first aid' section of the RLSS Handbook *Lifesaving*.

Material for Children and Young People

Although *Save A Life* is predominantly an adult education campaign, many instructors request information on training packages suitable for youngsters. The following materials may be useful but should, obviously, be pre-assessed by the teacher in the context of the class setting.

The St John Ambulance Three Cross Award – package including video cassette, *Emergency Aid in Schools* book, posters and certificates, etc.

Life Saving First Aid: Not Breathing; Bleeding Unconscious. These three booklets by Susan Foster and Ward Gardner are available from Kenneth Mason, Homewell, Havant, Hampshire as part of the *Keep Well* programme for infant and first school children. Slides film or video from Camera Talks Ltd.

The Royal Life Saving Society produces a 'Blue Code' for Water Safety leaflet aimed at young people and a 'Water Safety Resource Pack' for teachers of water safety. Both are available from the address opposite.

A Call for Help is a videofilm describing how to use the 999 telephone system to call an ambulance available from

Video Communication Services
Northampton Health Authority (Dept of Community Medicine)
c/o 39 Billing Road, Northampton, NN1 5BB
Tel: 0604 37853

REFERENCES, SOURCES AND FURTHER READING

First Aid and Resuscitation Standards, Guidebooks and Reference Texts

American Heart Association. Standards and guidelines for cardiopulmonary resuscitation and emergency cardiac care. *Journal of the American Medical Association* **255**, No. 21, 2841–3044, 1986.
First Aid. Combined manual of the St John Ambulance, British Red Cross Society and St Andrew's Ambulance Association, 1982, 4th edn., 2nd impr.
Resuscitation for the citizen. From the Resuscitation Council, UK, Dept of Anaesthetics, Royal Postgraduate Medical School, Hammersmith Hospital, Du Cane Road, London W12 0HS. Tel: 01-749 9974.
RESUSCITATION COUNCIL UK *The ABC of resuscitation*. British Medical Journal Publications, 1986.

History of Resuscitation

DEBARD, M. L. The history of cardiopulmonary resuscitation. *Annals of Emergency Medicine* **9** : 273–275, 1980.
HAWKINS, L. H. The history of resuscitation. *British Journal of Hospital Medicine* **4** : 495–500, 1970.
HEARNE, T. Elisha's child: theories in the history of CPR. *Emergency Medical Services Quarterly* **1** : 5–16, 1980.
JULIAN, D. G. Cardiac resuscitation in the 18th century. *Heart and Lung* **4** : 46–49, 1975.
PAYNE, J. P. On the resuscitation of the apparently dead. *Annals of the Royal College of Surgeons of England* **45** : 98–107, 1969.

Resuscitation Techniques

GORDON, A. S., FAINER, D. C. and IVY, A. C. Artificial respiration. A new method and a comparative study of different methods in adults. *Journal of the American Medical Association* **144**: 1455–1464, 1950.

JUDE, J. R., KOUWENHOVEN, W. B. and KNICKERBOCKER, G. G. Cardiac arrest: Report of applications of external cardiac massage on 118 patients. *Journal of the American Medical Association* **178**: 1063–1070, 1961.

KOUWENHOVEN, W. B., JUDE, J. R. and KNICKERBOCKER, G. G. Closed chest cardiac massage. *Journal of the American Medical Association* **173**: 1064–1067, 1960.

SAFAR, P. The failure of manual artificial respiration. *Journal of Applied Physiology* **14**: 84–88, 1959.

SAFAR, P., ESCARRAGA, L. and ELAM, J. O. A comparison of the mouth-to-mouth and mouth-to-airway methods of artificial respiration with the chest pressure arm-lift methods. *New England Journal of Medicine* **258**: 671–677, 1958.

Sudden Death and Community Training in Resuscitation

CUMMINS, R. O. and EISENBERG, M. S. Cardiopulmonary resuscitation. American style. *British Medical Journal* **291**: 1401–1403, 1985.

EISENBERG, M. S., BERGNER, L. and HALLSTROM, A. P. *Sudden cardiac death in the community* New York: Praeger, 1984.

LUND, I. and SKULBERG, A. Cardiopulmonary resuscitation by lay people. *Lancet* **ii**: 702–704, 1976.

LUND, I. and SKULBERG, A. Cardiopulmonary resuscitation in the street. *Lancet* **ii**: 1315–1318, 1982.

MARSDEN, A. K. Save a life: Profile of a community CPR campaign. *First Response* (Vitalograph House Journal) **1** (2), 1984.

THOMPSON, R. G., HALLSTROM, A. P. and COBB, L. A. Bystander initiated CPR in the management of ventricular fibrillation. *Annals of Internal Medicine* **90**: 737–740, 1978.

VINCENT, R., MARTIN, B. *et al*. A community training scheme in cardiopulmonary resuscitation. *British Medical Journal* **288**: 617–620, 1984.

Special Situations

ADDY, D. P. The choking child: back bangers against front pushers. *British Medical Journal* **286**: 536–537, 1983. (See also correspondence **286**: 721, 980.)

HARRIES, M. G. Drowning and near-drowning, fact and fiction. *Basic Journal* 7: 16–17, 1984.

The Heimlich manoeuvre (letter). *British Medical Journal* **286**: 1349–1350, 1983.

ZIDEMAN, D. A. Resuscitation in infants and children. (ABC of resuscitation series) *British Medical Journal*, **292**: 1584–1588.

Education

GATHERER, A., PARFIT, J. *et al. Is health education effective?* Health Education Council, 1979.

ROGERS, J. *Adults learning*, Open University Press, 1977.

ROGERS, J. *Adults in education*, BBC Publications, 1984.

Teaching Resuscitation

CAROLINE, N. L. *Life-supporting resuscitation and first aid – a manual for instructors of the lay public.* World Federation of Societies of Anaesthesiologists and League of Red Cross Societies, 1981.

You can save a life (CPR Instructors' Guide) Laerdal Medical, 1984. (Part of the group trainer from Laerdal.)

Acquired Immune Deficiency Syndrome

Aids: General information for doctors. DHSS, 1985.

NEWMAN, M. CPR and Aids: no known link. Special report. *Journal of the Emergency Medical Services* **Jan**: 83–84, 1986.

'Recommendations for decontaminating manikins used in cardiopulmonary resuscitation training (1983 update). Centers for Disease Control, Hepatitis Surveillance Report no. **42**: 34–36. American Heart Association and American Red Cross. (Updated in current *JAMA* 'standards', 1986.)

INDEX